YOUR BRAIN ON PLANTS

YOUR BRAIN ON PLANTS

Improve the Way You Think and Feel with Safe— and Proven—Medicinal Plants and Herbs

NICOLETTE PERRY, PhD,
and ELAINE PERRY, PhD

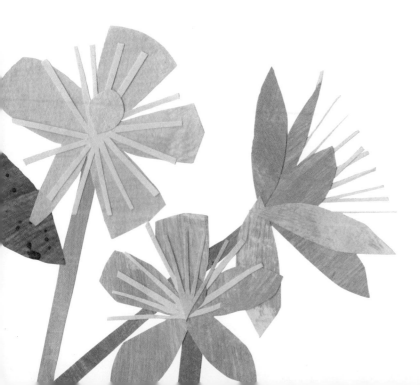

THE EXPERIMENT

NEW YORK

The Experiment, LLC
220 East 23rd Street, Suite 600
New York, NY 10010-4658
theexperimentpublishing.com

Many of the designations used by manufacturers and sellers to distinguish their products are claimed as trademarks. Where those designations appear in this book and The Experiment was aware of a trademark claim, the designations have been capitalized.

The Experiment's books are available at special discounts when purchased in bulk for premiums and sales promotions as well as for fund-raising or educational use. For details, contact us at info@theexperimentpublishing.com.

Library of Congress Cataloging-in-Publication Data

Names: Perry, Nicolette, author. | Perry, E. K. (Elaine K.) author.
Title: Your brain on plants : improve the way you think and feel with
    safe--and proven--medicinal plants and herbs / Nicolette Perry and Elaine
    Perry.
Other titles: Botanical brain balms
Description: New York : The Experiment, 2018. | "Originally published in UK
    as Botanical brain balms by Filbert Press in 2018"--Title page verso. |
    Includes bibliographical references and index.
Identifiers: LCCN 2017060581 (print) | LCCN 2018001843 (ebook) | ISBN
    9781615194476 (ebook) | ISBN 9781615194469 (pbk.)
Subjects: LCSH: Materia medica, Vegetable. | Medicinal plants. |
    Herbs--Therapeutic use.
Classification: LCC RC483 (ebook) | LCC RC483 .P45 2018 (print) | DDC
    615.7/88--dc23
LC record available at https://lccn.loc.gov/2017060581

ISBN 978-1-61519-446-9
Ebook ISBN 978-1-61519-447-6

Cover and text design by Sarah Smith
Illustrations by Clover Robin

Manufactured in China

First printing August 2018
10 9 8 7 6 5 4 3 2 1

To Ahau Chamahez, the Mayan god of medicine and good health

An Important Note to Readers

"Look to the nervous system as the key to maximum health."

—Galen

Contents

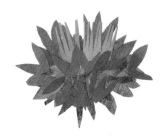

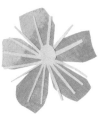

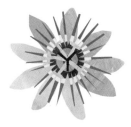

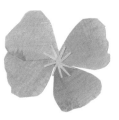

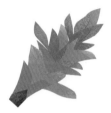
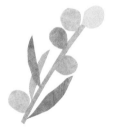
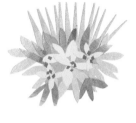
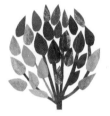

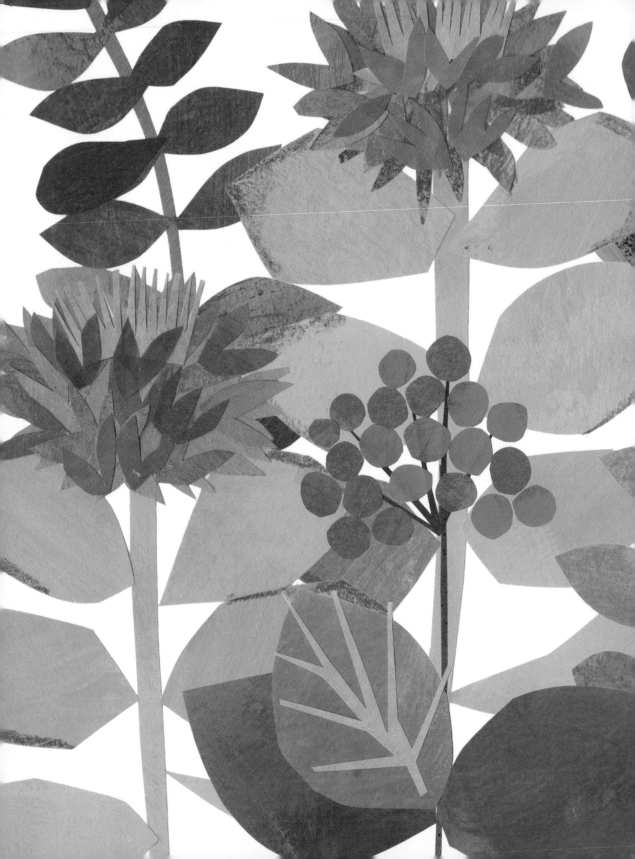

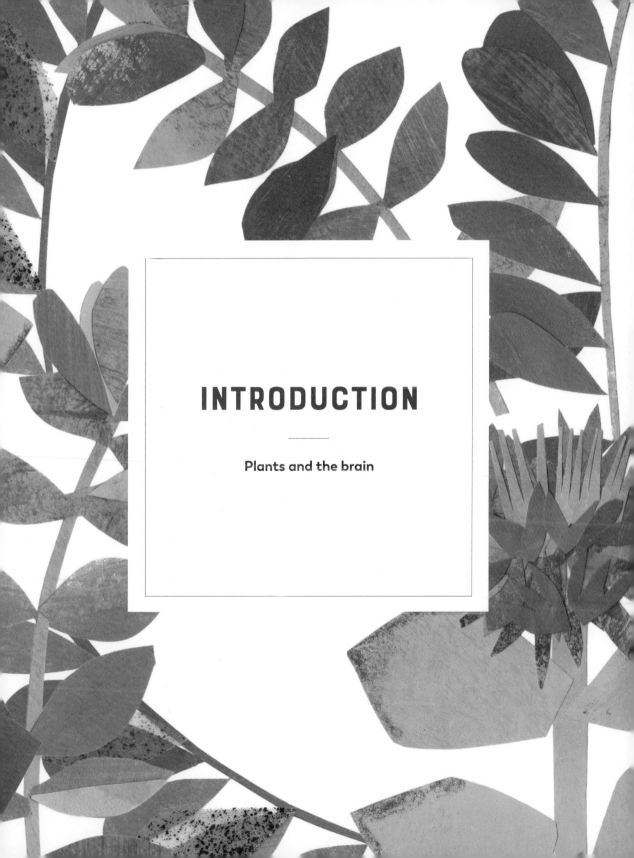

INTRODUCTION

Plants and the brain

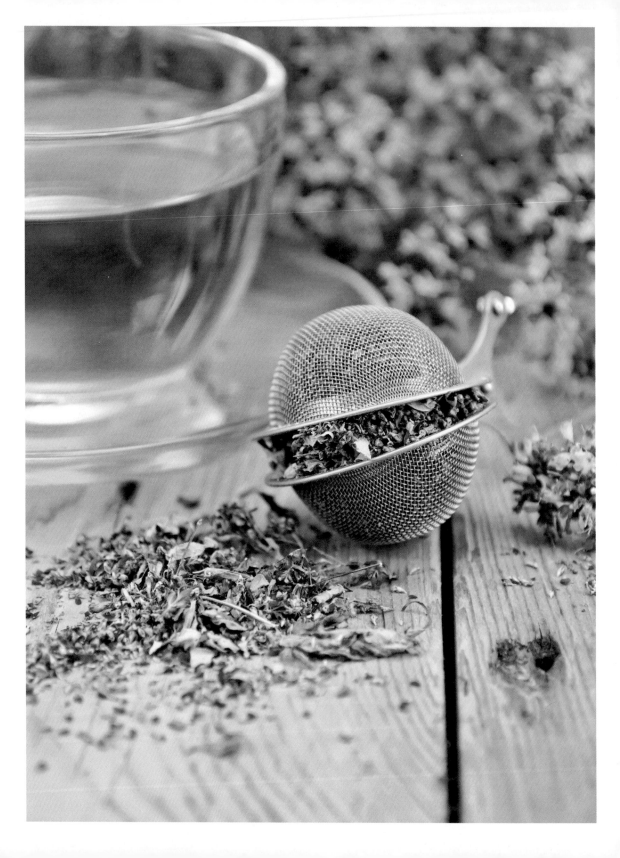

Whatever might prompt you to turn to plants for health, you are not alone. Since the beginning of the twenty-first century, annual sales of botanical supplements have doubled in the UK and the worldwide market for herbal products is now over $60 billion per annum.Scientific research on how plants improve brain function is increasing exponentially.

A glance at the herbal teas section of the supermarket or health food store speaks volumes about how plants for health are now an integral part of our lives and it's not just vegetarians and vegans who are putting plants at the center of their diet—we all understand better how fruit, vegetables, and other plants improve our overall health and well-being.

Taking plants for health is not new; it's just that we're starting to understand more about it. As early as the first century Hippocrates said, "Let food be thy medicine and medicine by thy food" and in 1906 Okakura Kakuzo wrote in *The Book of Tea* "tea began as a medicine and grew into a beverage." Science now shows that tea (*Camellia sinensis*) is just one of many ancient and traditionally used plants that enhance mental ability. A diet rich in plant foods, prepared to retain their bioactive compounds, has immediate effects on brain signaling and longer-term protective effects such as controlling inflammation, oxidation, and even protein deposits that accumulate in the aging brain. Although long-term benefits await clinical trials, there is convincing evidence that the Mediterranean diet, curry consumption, and drinking fruit juice reduce cognitive decline in groups that consume them. Whether as a food, spice, tincture, or capsule, there are many ways to get bioactive botanicals to your brain as preventative medicines, to enhance brain function, or to treat a condition.

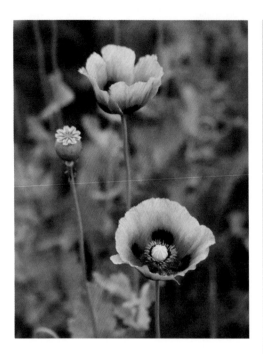

PLANTS AND THE BRAIN

With more than 100 brain signals, 100 billion brain cells, hundreds of trillions of connections and electrical currents traveling at up to 300 miles (483 km) per hour it's amazing the networks in the human brain work so well . . . most of the time.

Our aim is not just to tell you which plants work in the brain but to explain how and why they work. Understanding the individual ingredients of plants is the key to discovering how they enhance or nurture the brain. We're all familiar with the idea that plants provide our bodies with nutrition but less well known is the fact that many plants also contain chemicals that reach our brain cells and affect different pathways linked to being calm, sleeping well, and feeling positive. They do this by increasing or reducing neuron activity, more specifically mimicking, boosting, or blocking transmitter signals between brain cells.

Plant chemicals such as pain-relieving morphine from the opium poppy, stimulating caffeine from the coffee plant, and sedative cannabidiol in cannabis all work this way. Saffron, the "mellow yellow" from India and the Mediterranean, boosts the mood-lifting serotonin signal as effectively as SSRIs (selective serotonin reuptake inhibitors) for depression. European sage enhances the brain's memory signal acetylcholine, which earns it a place in Chapter 2: Cognition Boosters. Certain chemicals present in a number of plants are important to overall brain health. They maintain and protect neurons by controlling damage due to inflammation or oxidation, or by enhancing neuron growth.

WHY TAKE BOTANICAL BRAIN BALMS?

Botanical brain balms work in a different way from conventional medicine because plant extracts are "multidrugs," which means they contain a range of ingredients, each with different health benefits, unlike single-drug medicines. This means they can work on more than one aspect of the brain to beneficial effect.

Plant medicines are recognized by the highest authority. The World Health Organization (WHO) recognizes the use of herbal medicine in developing (and increasingly developed) countries as an essential component of primary health care. Doctors and pharmacists in parts of Europe prescribe plant medicine alongside mainstream medicine, for example St. John's wort for depression. Traditional plant medicines, as long as they are produced, prescribed, and used correctly, have a long legacy of safe use simply because they have been taken for hundreds if not thousands of years.

Most plant medicines have fewer side effects compared to pharmaceutical drugs,

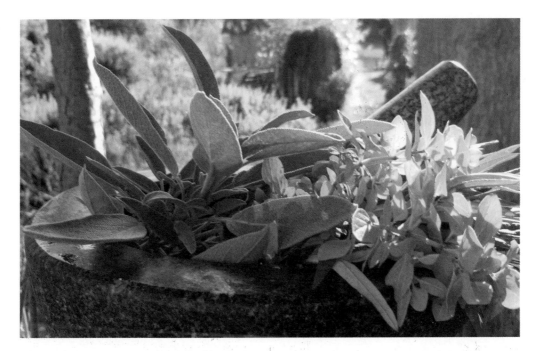

and some have none at all. Plant medicines are generally pleasant to take, and interspersed between the plant descriptions you'll find suggestions for making soothing or stimulating teas, muffins stuffed full of beneficial plants, a hops pillow to help you sleep, an aromatic room spray, or a happy face cream. One thing is for sure, plant extracts are a lot more agreeable to make part of your daily life than some prescription drugs for minor ailments and for long-term use as protectives.

MULTIDRUG PLANTS

Botanical brain balms are polypharmaceutical in the sense that multiple chemicals in them have additive actions and these offer advantages compared with single-chemical drugs. A range of chemicals in the antidepressant St. John's wort act on multiple brain signals to boost mood as well as to decrease inflammation and pain. In a controlled trial, compounds in cocoa (methylxanthines such as theobromine and caffeine) enhanced the beneficial effects of cocoa flavonoids on cardiovascular function. And combining plants has added effects— piperine in black pepper enhances the bioavailability of the blues-busting turmeric chemical (curcumin) by 2,000 percent.

Of course there are also good reasons to take a single plant chemical or drug. Standardization of complex chemical ingredients is not an issue (as in whole plant extracts) and dose is easy to regulate. Half of new drugs over the last thirty years come from plants, including leading treatments for pain, dementia, malaria, and cancer. So if you prefer to take your medicine as a chemical pill you can look forward to the development of new drugs from some of the brain balms described in this book.

Opposite: *Papaver somniferum* (opium poppy) contains pain-relieving morphine.
Above: Botanical brain balms freshly picked from Dilston Physic Garden.

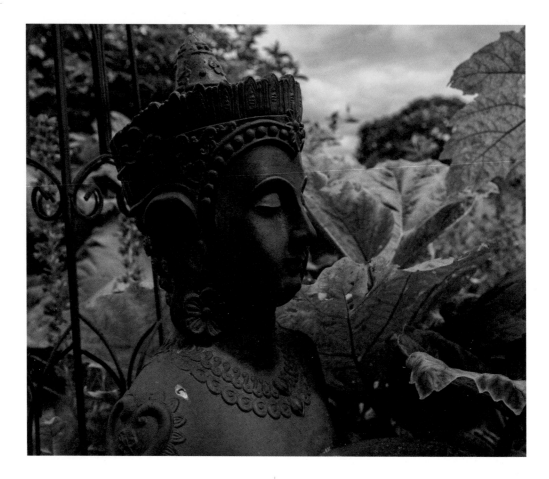

THE DILSTON EFFECT

The focus of this book is on plants that have positive effects on our mental health, and we are excited by the increasing scientific evidence to support the effects of plants on the mind and brain. For us it began with our university studies, conducted together with a team of neuroscientists, pharmacologists, and clinicians, in the pioneering years of the 1990s when research into plant medicine began in earnest. Today our research into plants for improving memory, attention, and mood continues at Dilston Physic Garden where we collaborate with medical herbalists, universities, the Royal Botanic Gardens, Kew, and research bodies to widen knowledge and understanding.

From the early days in the 1990s, people have visited Dilston Physic Garden to learn more about beneficial plants, appreciate them in their natural setting, and enjoy a uniquely restorative environment. With this book, we wanted to share a little of that Dilston effect whether you're looking for a gentle pick-me-up or relief from a particular symptom.

In these pages you will find detailed profiles on fifty-six plants that we have carefully selected as our top plants for mind and mood on the basis of their performance in clinical trials. We've included other plants that are well

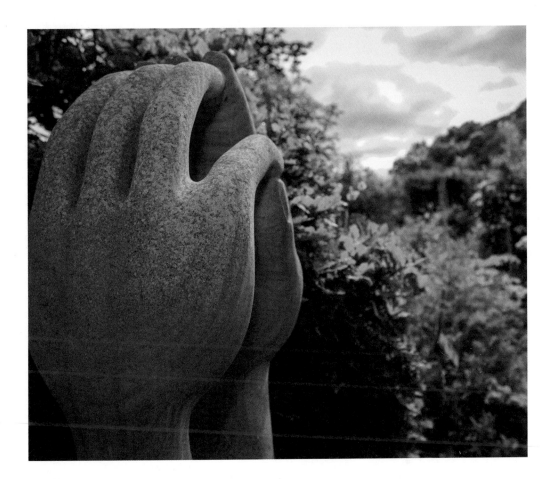

supported by traditional use and laboratory tests, and these may be the ones to watch for the future.

HOW TO USE THE BOOK

The fifty-six plants selected for inclusion are grouped into chapters, and in Chapters 1 through 5 they are listed according to the weight of their scientific evidence, those with the most science behind them first. This ranking has not been applied to the Extra Energizers in Chapter 6 because scientific evidence for "mental fatigue" and "lack of vitality" is harder to establish. The mind-altering plants in Chapter 7 are listed in order of mildest to strongest. And

finally, the all-rounders in Chapter 8 have not been ranked because their effects are so wide ranging it's impossible to draw comparisons.

Each chapter opens with an explanation of how the plants and their constituents affect the brain, and the key mechanisms involved. Along with the lead plants, there are additional descriptions of plants that have been used traditionally for hundreds of years and plants that are becoming the focus of scientific scrutiny and some way along the process of gaining recognition.

Above and following pages: Visitors come to Dilston Physic Garden to learn more about beneficial plants, appreciate them in their natural setting, and enjoy a uniquely restorative environment.

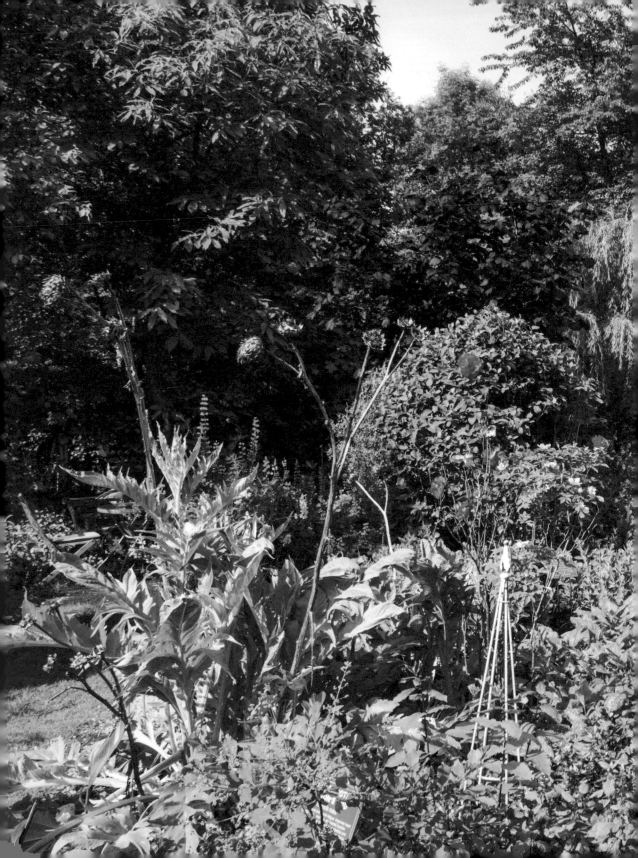

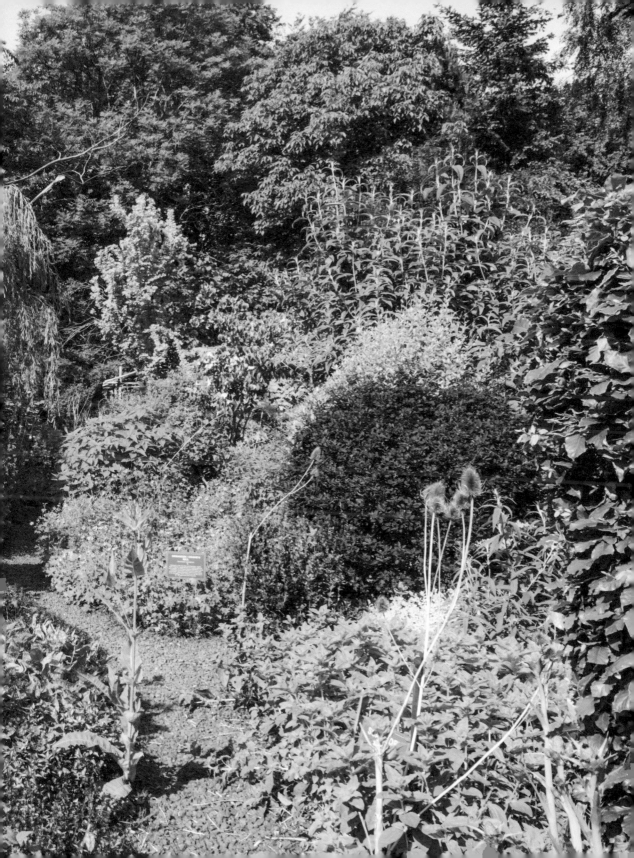

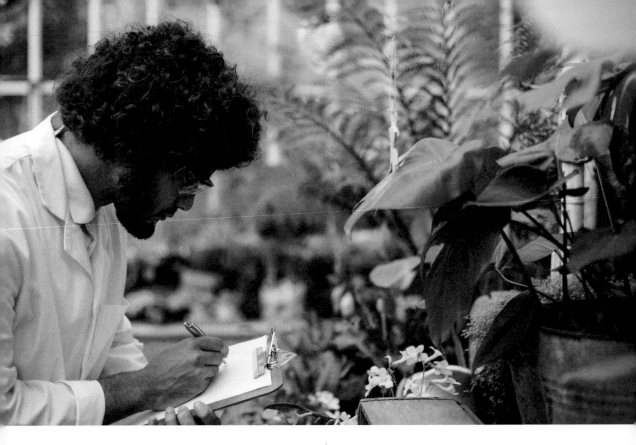

PLANT ENTRY

Beneath each plant entry you will find the following information.

- A photo of the plant for identification purposes.
- The common name of the plant preceded by the all-important botanical name, which is the one to rely on when it comes to correct identification of the plant.
- A short description of the key health benefits of the plant.

ABOUT THE PLANT

Describes the key physical characteristics of the plant, its native origins, preferred growing environment and information about different parts of the plant.

HISTORY AND FOLKLORE

Wherever they live, people have always used the plants that grow around them; for example, calming passionflower is widely used in South America. A long period of traditional use provides important information about the plant's safe use and effects on the central nervous system. For example, St. John's wort, a well-known plant for mild depression, is also known as "chase devil," referring back to the Middle Ages when depression was thought to be caused by spirit possession.

Above: Research into plants that improve memory, attention and mood continues and plants used traditionally for centuries are often the focus for scientific research.
Opposite: *Salvia officinalis* (European sage) was included in lab tests by the authors because of its long-standing reputation in old herbals for helping memory.

WHAT SCIENTISTS SAY

Scientific backing is the starting point for a plant to be listed in full in the book, and reflects the way we work. How do we decide that a plant has passed the mark on scientific evidence? Chemistry and lab studies help to explain how the plant works, but human studies are essential, as for any pharmaceutical. In human studies, controlled clinical trials are the "gold standard." Robust reviews and meta-analysis of multiple trials for modern medicines confirm the value of plants such as arnica for mild pain and St. John's wort to improve mood.

KEY INGREDIENTS

The plant ingredients that impact on the brain are "secondary metabolites," chemicals produced by the plant to sustain its health in its environment that happen to benefit our health, too, and not the plant food ingredients concerned with nutrition such as proteins, fats, minerals, and vitamins. The main known bioactive ingredients are highlighted for each plant, though any single plant can contain from 40 to 200 or more chemicals and some can work synergistically. Chemical content and ratios can vary according to where the plant is grown (altitude, soil type, hours of sunlight for example) and variations in single chemicals of up to 20 percent are reported.

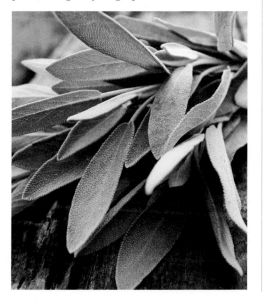

Familiar plant chemicals such as flavonoids in blueberries sit alongside those that are less familiar like cineole from sage and juglone from walnuts.

Many of the plants in this book provide benefits beyond the brain. Some act on circulation, metabolism, and digestive systems essential for optimal brain function such as metabolic (antidiabetes) and cardiovascular benefits. Where these effects are prominent they are included. These plants have many other bodily effects such as being key antivirals and antibacterials (even farmers are turning to them to keep animals healthy in the face of bacterial resistance to conventional antibiotics).

HOW TO TAKE IT

Dose indicates one or more of the common methods of taking the plant and is in the range recommended by medical herbalists. Doses have been checked as far as possible to be consistent with those used in clinical trials, which report the safety as well as efficacy of the plant. These are very broad guidelines, and plant effects can vary with individuals depending on their weight, age, diet, and clinical history, and the formulation. Consult an authoritative herbal medicine book or a registered medical herbalist for precise dose, or if purchased take as per product instructions.

Some plants can be used safely at normal levels for foodstuffs while others are specific to a condition and should only be taken at the recommended dose—unwanted side effects can occur at incorrect dose levels. Medical herbalists frequently start a patient at a lower dose for certain plant medicines and indicate they may take time to act (and some say the longer a symptom or condition has lasted, the longer the plant will take to act). Other plants can be rapid onset, such as peppermint for pain, valerian and hop for sleep.

For each plant the standard or most popular way to take the plant is given, whether this is tea, tincture, capsule, or tablet. If a plant is eaten as a foodstuff we say so. The best way to take a plant can depend on the most effective method to get active ingredients to the brain. Ensure you are familiar with the different methods of taking plants by reading "How to use the book" (page 7) and the glossary (page 202).

It is possible to grow medicinal plants in much the same way as you grow fruits and vegetables. Make sure you grow the correct plant by checking the botanical name, use the correct plant parts, harvest at the correct times (when active plant chemicals are at their highest), dry within 7 to 10 days in aerated conditions and out of sunlight, and store in a dark paper bag, loosely sealed to avoid fungal and bacterial growth. Variability in concentration of constituents can occur, and there is some evidence that plants grown organically may contain more bioactive ingredients.

Below: Many of the brain balms in this book can be grown at home and harvested for drying. Store in dark paper bags in a cool, dry place.

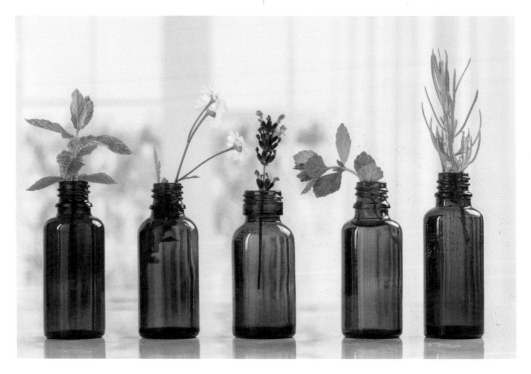

SAFETY

Safety advice specific to the plant is provided here but it's also important to read the disclaimer on page vi. Knowledge and best practice in plant medicine and pharmacology are constantly changing and as new research is carried out, as in mainstream medicine, contraindications with other medicines will also change. Always consult a registered medical herbalist or your health care provider for the latest information if you are pregnant, on any medication, or have any condition.

Consulting a medical herbalist and/or pharmacist is the best way to find out which plants may be best for you especially if your usual health care provider is not an expert. Education and associated guidance on the use of plants vary from country to country. In Asia, use of plant medicine is mainstream; in the Middle East and some European countries, doctors and pharmacists prescribe or recommend plant as well as drug medicines; and in the US and UK plant medicine is not yet mainstream, and a registered practitioner in herbal medicine should be consulted. Choose a qualified medical herbalist or other practitioner (in aromatherapy, yoga, or tai chi, for example) who has the relevant education, professional membership, and insurance. You can also obtain reliable information on safe plants to take at home from authoritative online sources and handbooks.

Important regulations with regard to the plant's use may also be listed here.

Below: Chamomile is one of the oldest known medicinal plants and a popular herbal tea to promote sleep and relieve anxiety.

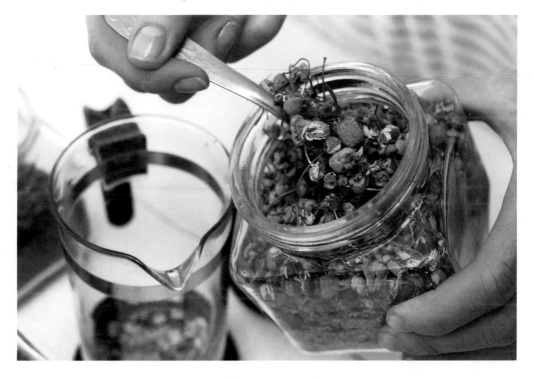

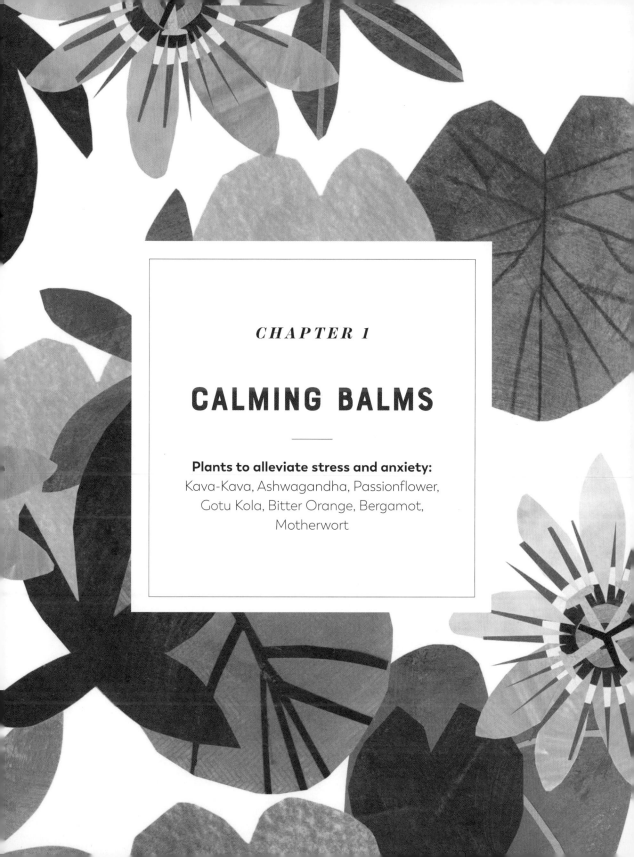

CHAPTER 1

CALMING BALMS

Plants to alleviate stress and anxiety:
Kava-Kava, Ashwagandha, Passionflower,
Gotu Kola, Bitter Orange, Bergamot,
Motherwort

Each day, more and more people fall victim to the twenty-first century's anxiety epidemic and many of them are prescribed orthodox treatments that focus on the antianxiety drug benzodiazepine or antidepressant drugs such as the SSRIs (selective serotonin reuptake inhibitors) that can have undesirable side effects such as drowsiness, addiction, or cognitive impairment. Keeping us calm is just one of the many wonderful things plants can do for our brains whether we need a light stress reliever or something more serious. And there are many plant-based remedies that are scientifically proven to induce calm and reduce anxiety, tension, and stress without unwelcome side effects. Reassuringly, science is now able to show exactly how these plant medicines work by acting on neurotransmitters—the brain chemicals that relay signals from one brain cell to another.

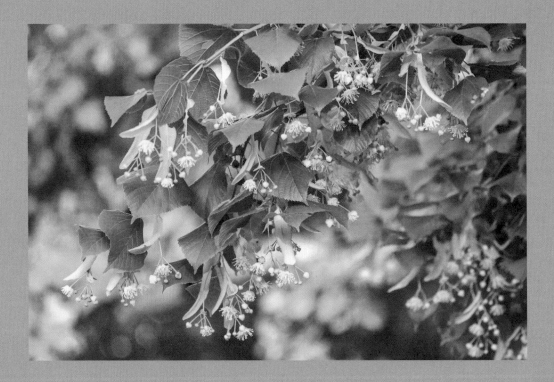

HOW DO CALMING BALMS WORK?

Calming balms often influence a brain signal called GABA (gamma-aminobutyric acid) where antianxiety drugs (benzodiazepines) are also effective. GABA prevents brain cells from firing too often and is essentially the brain's main decelerator or calming signal. Some plant ingredients can prolong GABA's effect in the brain while others can mimic or boost its calming action. There are also plant ingredients that enhance the mood-boosting (serotonin) signal, and others that block the main signal that excites or stimulates (glutamate). It's likely that there are plants that have still to reveal brain mechanisms we are not yet aware of, just as the opium poppy led to the discovery of a whole new raft of brain signals, the endorphins.

THE TRANQUILITY PLANTS

For this chapter we have selected seven lead plants, some of which have the "gold standard" backing in medical science. The calming South Seas kava-kava is followed by the sedative tonic ashwagandha and Ayurvedic calmer gotu kola. Also included are edible fruits—passionflower, bitter orange, bergamot—and finally motherwort, which has been used in Europe since the sixteenth century. Some of these calming balms are also mildly sleep inducing, with ashwagandha and passionflower recognized for their sedative properties. Traditional use of these plants extends back hundreds if not thousands of years and still informs twenty-first-century scientific research into calming botanicals.

There are many other calming plants, such as holy basil (*Ocimum tenuiflorum*) and lime (linden) blossom (*Tilia cordata*), which are firmly established in herbal medicine and have some scientific support but are yet to be examined for their calming effects in humans.

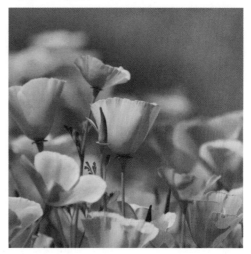

Some of these get a mention during the course of the chapter.

Then there are other wonderful brain balms that have a range of therapeutic benefits that include but are not limited to calming—chamomile, lemon balm, lavender, skullcap, valerian, hops, California poppy, and vervain. Find out about these in later chapters.

ABOUT CALMING BALMS AT DILSTON

Our research into calming plants began when we received a funding award from the Mental Health Foundation to research plant therapy for people with dementia. One of the criteria was that the research had to concentrate on complementary medicine, a tough brief at the time for our conventional science team. We hit on the idea of an aromatherapy-based clinical trial using essential oils, taken from traditional plants, to calm older people with dementia. Some people with this condition become anxious and agitated and are treated with drugs (neuroleptics) designed to control

Opposite: Calming *Tilia cordata* (lime), firmly established in herbal medicine and with some scientific support.
Above: *Eschscholzia californica* (California poppy) has a range of therapeutic benefits including calming.

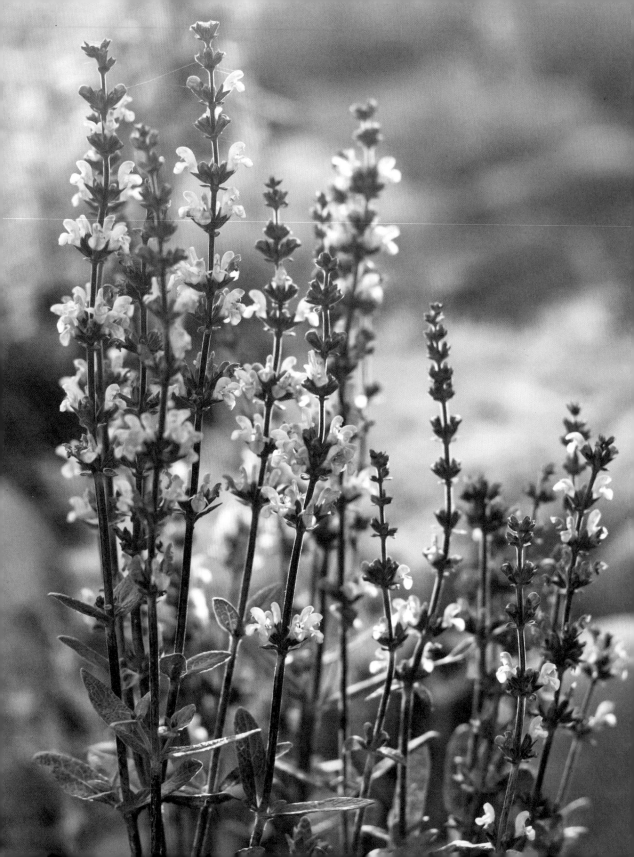

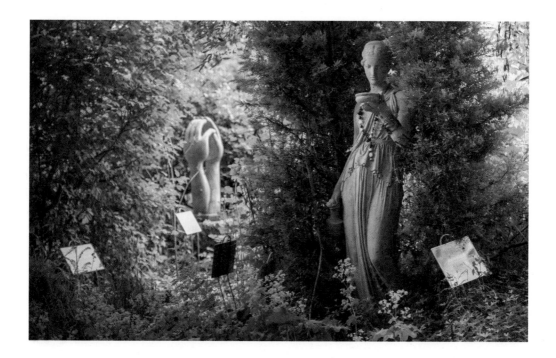

the behavioral problems this generates, but these drugs sedate and lead to tremors, potentially dangerous falls, and even cognitive impairment. Our first clinical trial, which used lemon balm (*Melissa officinalis*), was surprisingly successful.

Ten years later we still have plans to initiate research on new plants with calming properties, and below we list the seven calming balms proven by science to have safe use for resolving stress and keeping anxiety at bay. We have listed them according to the weight of their scientific backing—those with the most science behind them first.

Opposite: *Verbena officinalis* (vervain) is traditionally used to relieve tension, anxiety, long-term stress, and exhaustion.
Above: Research into calming balms at Dilston Physic Garden began with an aromatherapy-based clinical trial using essential oils taken from traditional plants.

TRADITIONAL CALMERS

Keeping anxiety at bay is a universal necessity. In many parts of the world people have used their local plant medicines for hundreds of years to help relieve anxiety, and continue to do so. Some of these plants are undergoing the first steps in rigorous scientific exploration and it is encouraging to see the list growing. Many may be found to contain the same chemical ingredients that are responsible for calming effects attributed to scientifically backed plants. For example, coriander (*Coriandrum sativum*), lavender (*Lavandula* species), and clary sage (*Salvia sclarea*) contain the aromatic ingredient linalool, which blocks our brain signal that excites (glutamate), enhances our mood-boosting signal (serotonin) and has similar antianxiety benefits to diazepam.

UNDER INVESTIGATION

The following plants have not yet been fully

explored by science but enjoy the backing of a modest amount of evidence: holy basil (*Ocimum tenuiflorum*), Japanese cedar (*Cryptomeria japonica*), European oats (*Avena sativa*), fennel (*Foeniculum vulgare*), celery (*Apium graveolens*), pasqueflower (*Pulsatilla vulgaris*), white waterlily (*Nymphaea alba*), stachys (*Stachys lavandulifolia*), fenugreek (*Trigonella foenum-graecum*), date plum (*Diospyros lotus*), mountain thistle (*Acanthus montanus*), tuberose (*Polianthes tuberosa*), coneflower (*Echinacea* species), Jamaican dogwood (*Piscidia piscipula*), and cramp bark (*Viburnum opulus*).

Below: *Pulsatilla vulgaris* (pasqueflower) and *Foeniculum vulgare* (fennel) **opposite** have not yet been fully explored but there's some scientific evidence of their calming properties.

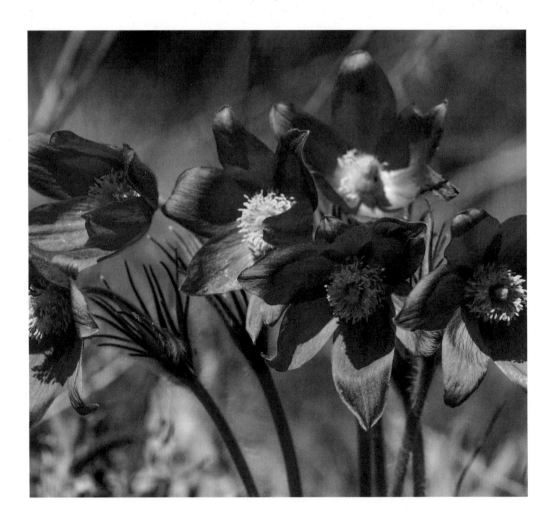

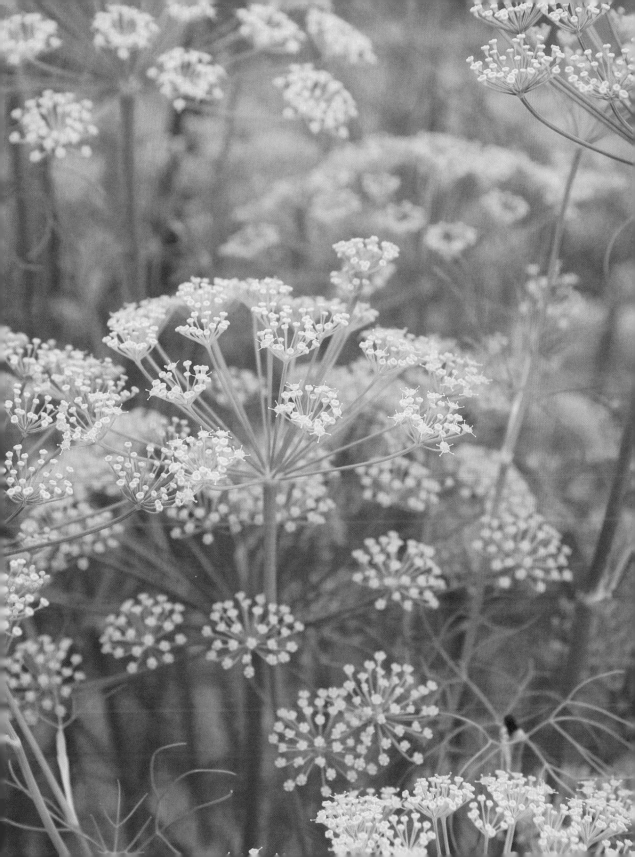

Piper methysticum

KAVA-KAVA

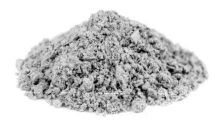

Famous South Seas ritual calming tonic with a mass of clinical evidence behind it to support its effectiveness for treating anxiety and nervous tension. As it relaxes body and mind while maintaining mental acuity, it is the plant to take when you need to be calm but also stay alert.

ABOUT THE PLANT: This evergreen climbing shrub from the pepper family grows to 33 feet (10 m) with sparse branches, large, heart-shaped leaves, and a thin green spike as a flower. Within the South Sea islands it grows as far east as Hawaii, and it is now cultivated in the USA and Australia. Propagated from runners, it's the dried root, harvested at any time of the year, that is most used. As a drink it's sweet, hot, and bitter, without much odor, and leaves the mouth slightly numb. It's closely related to the stimulant *Piper sanctum*.

HISTORY AND FOLKLORE: Also called awa in Hawaii, where it arrived in sailing canoes from the Polynesian islands a thousand years ago, kava is noted mainly for its ability to calm and relax. It's been used for thousands of years as a drink with antianxiety effects similar to drinking wine because it delivers "a relaxed, sociable state where fatigue and anxiety are lessened and eventually give a deep restful sleep, from which the user awakens refreshed without a hangover" (according to medical herbalists Kerry Bone and Simon Mills). In excessive quantities it's said to produce a euphoric state and is used (traditionally, chewed and fermented with saliva) by Pacific Islanders in ceremonies to communicate with gods. It's also used traditionally as a mental stimulant, euphoric, and aphrodisiac, for local pain relief, and to treat teething and restlessness in children.

WHAT SCIENTISTS SAY

In humans: Many controlled clinical trials indicate kava's efficacy in reducing anxiety, restlessness and nervous tension. It's nonaddictive and said to be nonhypnotic. German and French studies show it doesn't have sedative effects and doesn't undermine the ability to drive. Shown by clinical trials to be comparable to orthodox antianxiety (benzodiazepine) and antidepressant drugs, it also improves alertness, memory, and reaction time. Clinical studies show its benefits as a treatment for mild depression, sleep disturbances, epilepsy, menopause, and local pain relief.

In Ludwig-Maximilians University in Germany an eight-week multicenter controlled trial showed kava to be as effective and safe as the antidepressant opipramol and the antianxiety drug buspirone in the acute treatment of generalized anxiety disorder in 129 people.

In the lab: Studies show it boosts the brain's calming (GABA) signal. It also enhances the brain's pleasure and reward signals (serotonin, dopamine, noradrenaline, and cannabinoid), affects pain signals, and is anti-inflammatory and neuroprotective.

KEY INGREDIENTS: A resin that has kava lactones such as kavain and yangonin which are anti-anxiety, relaxant (antispasmodic) and have local anaesthetic effects. Kavain in particular is calming and shown to be as effective as a benzodiazepine. Alkaloids such as pipermethystine.

HOW TO TAKE IT: Root tea 4 to 6 g dried (8 to 12 g fresh) per 500 ml water per day. Capsules, tinctures, and powders are also taken.

SAFETY: Safe in moderate doses but not recommended by some for prolonged period (over 3 months). Do not use in pregnancy, liver disorder, or Parkinson's. Caution if taken with other sedative drugs and alcohol. Long term and high doses may eventually undermine skin health but this clears once treatment ends.

Regulated on account of concerns following bouts of unexplained hepatotoxicity of ethanolic extracts, but bans, for example in Germany, are being overturned because the cause of this short-term toxicity is not clear. (Some lab studies fail to show liver toxicity of ethanolic extract and individual alkaloids, and the rare cases of toxicity may have been due to overdose, prolonged use, adulteration, or a toxic mold contamination in harvesting and storage.)

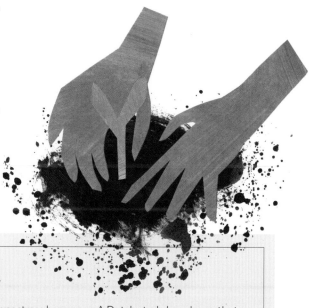

Garden yourself better

Being outdoors in the natural world can lower stress hormones. A Dutch study has shown that doing repetitive tasks such as gardening can also help to alleviate stress better than other less active leisure pursuits. In the study, one group was asked to read indoors after completing a stressful task while the other group gardened for 30 minutes. The gardeners reported being in a better mood than the readers, and also had lower levels of the stress hormone cortisol.

So why not get out in the garden? If you don't have your own, find one nearby where volunteers are welcome. Weeding or pruning will reduce feelings of stress and anxiety—and if you do grow a chamomile lawn, the weeding will provide the added bonus of a calming aroma.

Withania somnifera

ASHWAGANDHA

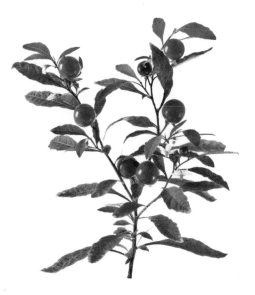

High-flying Indian Ayurvedic nerve tonic that calms, improves mental and physical health in nervous exhaustion, and enhances memory. A plant for when you need to be calm, rest, and reboot.

ABOUT THE PLANT: This shrub in the potato family likes dry places. Growing to 5 feet (1.5 m), it has oval leaves with greenish or vivid yellow flowers that turn into bright red berries. Native to Asia, Africa, and Europe, it now grows throughout the Middle East and Mediterranean. Its Hindi/Sanskrit name is *ashwagandha* but it is also known as Indian ginseng and withania. Leaves are harvested in spring and the berries and root in autumn; all parts of the plant are used.

HISTORY AND FOLKLORE: The Ancient Greek physician Dioscorides (c.40 to c.90 AD) advocated its use as a tonic, and it's been employed in Indian herbal medicine for centuries to calm and strengthen nerves, clear the mind, and promote restful sleep. *Somnifera* means "sleep-inducer" in Latin, a clue to its use as a mild sedative and calming plant. Ashwagandha means "horse smell" in Sanskrit, which refers to its strong odor and also relates to its "horse's strength" as a calming tonic. Its berries are chewed in India during recuperation from illness and to improve vitality and longevity. Those who are familiar with Chinese ginseng may know ashwagandha is used in much the same way to strengthen the nervous system, but note that ashwagandha is a mild sedative, whereas ginseng is a mild stimulant. Ashwagandha is also traditionally used for insomnia, to restore health in the elderly, slow down premature aging, delay senile debility, as an aphrodisiac, and as an adaptogen to support the treatment of chronic conditions (because it helps the body's stress systems adapt).

WHAT SCIENTISTS SAY

In humans: In India in the 1960s, ashwagandha alkaloids were identified as calming and sedative. In several controlled clinical trials it significantly lowered anxiety compared to a placebo, as well as reducing body stress symptoms such as blood pressure and heart rate and improving well-being scores. A controlled trial also found it to be a safe and effective aid in the treatment of obsessive compulsive disorder. It has become a widely studied medicinal plant, and pilot clinical trials show other restorative effects, such as the enhancement of cognitive skills and memory in bipolar disorder and lowering cardiovascular risk factors. It also improves conditions associated with aging such as loss of muscle strength and function, and pain in osteoarthritis, while also preventing anemia, promoting growth in children, improving stamina in athletes, and improving sexual function in women.

In the lab: Numerous studies confirm its action within our brain, where it modifies a range of neurotransmitters including those which calm (GABA), excite (glutamate), are antidepressant (serotonin), affect memory (acetylcholine), affect pain (opioid), and influence stress and immune (corticosterone) signals. Other potential brain benefits of this plant are its all-important antioxidant and anti-inflammatory properties as well as its contribution to blood-vessel growth and the protection of nerve cells.

KEY INGREDIENTS: Key bioactive ingredients of ashwagandha are triterpene withaferins and withanolides (steroidal lactones similar to our own steroid hormones), which were shown to be anti-inflammatory in the 1970s and also inhibit cancer cells. It contains active alkaloids and iron, too.

HOW TO TAKE IT: Root decoction 3 to 5 g per 200 ml water per day. Fresh leaves and berries and capsules of the root powder are also taken. Berries are used in cheese making as a substitute to coagulate milk.

SAFETY: No known side effects, contraindications, or special precautions. At high dose it may enhance benzodiazepine effects, be thyroid stimulating, or cause gastro upset.

Passiflora incarnata

PASSIONFLOWER

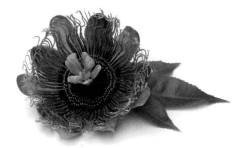

Effective calming plant with the most beautiful flowers. Used to soothe the mind, reduce anxiety, and also as a sedative for occasional insomnia. Its discovery as a medicine depended on a fascinating blend of native South American and Christian cultures.

ABOUT THE PLANT: A native of southeastern USA and Central and South America, this perennial climber is also cultivated in Europe. It has three-lobed, toothed leaves and large purple-blue flowers. Although hardy, *P. incarnata* needs a sheltered spot with plenty of sun. Gather when flowering or in fruit. Its yellow-orange fruits are the size of hens' eggs and are edible, although not as delicious as those familiar fruits from *Passiflora edulis*, which has also been investigated scientifically.

HISTORY AND FOLKLORE: Widely used by indigenous Americans for its calming and sleep-inducing effects. Some *Passiflora* species are used shamanically, added to ayuahuasca, an Amazonian plant mix used to promote altered states of consciousness. Spanish missionaries decided that the flower has a sacred geometry, based on the form and numbers of parts of the flower, which they thought reflected the last days of Christ, hence the name passionflower. Used in herbal medicine for anxiety, restlessness, irritability, and pain relief (premenstrual syndrome, dysmenorrhea, muscle cramps, neuralgia), and to promote pleasant dreams. Also as a peripheral vasodilator, for abnormal cardiac rhythm and to prevent tachycardia.

WHAT SCIENTISTS SAY

In humans: A number of controlled studies support passionflower's calming effects on the central nervous system. It reduces general anxiety as well as anxiety before anaesthesia, dental treatment, and surgery; reduces insomnia and improves the quality of sleep; and is successful in the management of opiate withdrawal.

It also lowers emotional and behavioral problems in anxious children. In controlled trials it has been shown useful for pain relief,

lowering insulin resistance in diabetes and for asthmatic symptoms.

In the lab: *P. incarnata* (and others in the genus such as *P. edulis*) affects a host of brain signals. It enhances calming (GABA) and affects excitatory (glutamate) pathways and its harmala alkaloids inhibit monoamine oxidase (associated with anti-depressive effects). Passionflower is antispasmodic, anticonvulsant and neuroprotective (via its ingredient isovitexin). It also affects the brain's pleasure (cannabinoid), pain (opioid) and memory (acetylcholine) signals.

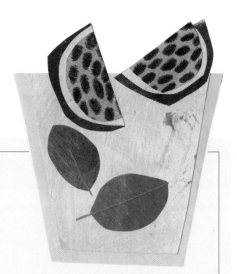

Passionfruit caipirinha

2 limes, cut in wedges
4 fresh lime leaves (optional)
2 passionfruit, cut in half
2 tablespoons light brown sugar
2 ounces (60 ml) vodka

Put the lime wedges, 2 lime leaves if using, pulp from 1 passionfruit, and sugar in a cocktail shaker. Muddle together with the end of rolling pin or a wooden spoon handle.
Stir in the vodka, add crushed ice, and shake or stir well.

Half-fill 2 tumblers with crushed ice and divide the unstrained caipirinha mixture between them.
Fill to the top with crushed ice and add 2 lime leaves and the remaining passionfruit halves.

In a controlled clinical trial at Tehran University in Iran, passionflower extract was as effective as a benzodiazepine in the treatment of generalized anxiety disorder and, unlike the benzodiazepine, reduced anxiety without impairing job performance.

KEY INGREDIENTS: Punjab University in India has been studying its ingredients since 2001. It contains the antianxiety flavonoid hesperidin (in citrus fruits such as bergamot and also in valerian), which also affects the brain signal where caffeine works (adenosine). It also contains the flavonoid luteolin (also in chamomile and lemon balm) and less common flavonoids such as orientin and schaftoside. Its small amounts of harmala alkaloids such as harmine (also present in ayahuasca) which show psychostimulant effects are not usually present in commercial samples. There may be two chemical types of *Passiflora*, those with isovitexin and schaftoside dominating and those with swertisin and low schaftoside.

HOW TO TAKE IT: Dried leaf tea 2 to 3 g (4 to 6 g fresh) per 240 ml water 2 times daily. Leaves, flowers, or powdered fruit peel, used in capsules, tablets, and tinctures are common over-the-counter remedies. It's difficult to beat the fresh fruit (also known as maypop as it pops if stood on), and fruit juice and curd may also be prepared.

SAFETY: Listed in the natural pharmacopoeias of France, Germany, and Switzerland. Extract is classified as "generally regarded as safe" (GRAS) by the Food and Drug Administration. Caution with benzodiazepines, sedatives, and monoamine oxidase inhibitors. Possible caution in cardiovascular disorders. Large doses can produce drowsiness.

Centella asiatica syn.
Hydrocotyle asiatica

GOTU KOLA

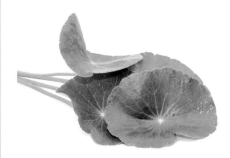

Gotu kola is another famous Ayurvedic relaxing plant with some science behind it. Known as a "panacea" calming medicine, it's said to rejuvenate and restore the mind, the body, and the spirit.

ABOUT THE PLANT: Also called Indian pennywort, centella, brahmi, and tsubo kusa (Japan). Native to India, it's now widespread through the tropics including the southern USA. Liking marshes and riversides, this evergreen perennial creeping herb has small round leaves and pale pink flowers. Aerial parts are harvested throughout the year and have an aromatic, spicy, sweet taste. Not to be confused with European marsh pennywort (*Hydrocotyle vulgaris*), which is not used therapeutically.

HISTORY AND FOLKLORE: Used in 3,000-year-old Ayurvedic medicine, and now in Western herbal medicine, as a rejuvenating plant to calm nerves, strengthen the nervous system and boost cognition. Some think the leaves look like the brain. This fits with the "doctrine of signatures" which supports the theory that a plant looks like what it's good for. It is known as the longevity herb—ancient texts talk of it prolonging life and being the herb of enlightenment. Apparently elephants like eating gotu.

WHAT SCIENTISTS SAY

In humans: In controlled clinical trials, gotu is so far shown to be effective in the treatment of generalized anxiety disorder and in reducing stress and anxiety against placebo. Also when tested in combination with three other plants, cognitive function in children improved over three months, and gotu was more effective than folic acid in improving cognitive function after stroke.

In the lab: Gotu works to enhance our calming (GABA) neurotransmitter and is also beneficial in sleep deprivation and depression models. It also helps memory by boosting the memory signal acetylcholine, shows protection against various brain diseases in lab models, and promotes neurone growth. On top of this it has the all-important brain dividend of being antioxidant and anti-inflammatory.

KEY INGREDIENTS: A key bioactive is asiatic acid, which lowers anxiety and depression and boosts the brain's memory signal acetylcholine. Contains saponins such as madecassoside and asiaticoside, which also lower anxiety; the latter has also been widely studied in skin healing. Its essential oil contains calming and cognition-boosting pinenes, humulene (also in sleep-promoting hops), and caryophyllene (also in cognition-boosting common sage). Also contains health-giving flavonoids, carotenoids, and vitamins B and C.

HOW TO TAKE IT: In India and other countries gotu is commonly eaten as a green leafy vegetable and the fresh leaves are used as a tonic herb in salads and juices. Also taken as a dried tea 2 to 5 g (or 4 to 10 g fresh) per 240 ml water, 35 ml 2 times daily. Tincture or capsules are easily mixed with food and drink as a general tonic.

SAFETY: Occasional allergic reaction, gastro upset, contact dermatitis, and may cause sensitivity to sunlight. No adverse effects seen at normal doses, though larger doses may cause vertigo. May reduce fertility. Not in pregnancy. Caution in liver disease, diabetes, and with sedative medication.

Bitter orange and almond cake (gluten-free)

Makes an 8-inch (20 cm) cake

FOR THE CAKE:

14 ounces (400 g) whole bitter
   (Seville) oranges, or canned Seville
   oranges prepared for marmalade
4 eggs
1 cup (225 g) superfine sugar or 6
   tablespoons (150 ml) honey
3 cups (250 g) ground almonds
2 teaspoons gluten-free baking
   powder
1 teaspoon chopped gotu kola leaves

FOR THE TOPPING:

3 drops neroli essential oil
3 tablespoons marmalade
2 whole sweet oranges (sliced) or
   candied bitter orange peel (sliced)

This moist cake uses bitter oranges to calm frayed
nerves, and the dense texture provided by the
ground almonds is comforting. If you are using
canned oranges, skip the first two steps and
measure out the required quantity.

1 Place the oranges in a large saucepan, cover with
cold water, and bring to a boil. Simmer for 2 hours,
drain, and cool.

2 Break open the oranges and remove the seeds, then
blitz the fruit in a food processor or blender.

3 Heat the oven to 375°F (190°C). Grease the base
and sides of an 8-inch (20 cm) springform pan and
line with parchment paper.

4 With a beater, whisk the eggs with the sugar or
honey until thick and foamy.

5 Mix together the ground almonds, baking powder,
pulped oranges, and gotu kola leaves, and then fold in
the beaten egg mixture.

6 Pour into the prepared cake pan and bake for 1
hour or until an inserted skewer comes out clean. You
may need to cover it after 35 minutes with aluminum
foil to prevent burning. Remove from the oven and
leave to cool on a wire rack.

7 When the cake is completely cool, add the neroli
essential oil to the marmalade and spread a thin layer
over the top of the cake. Decorate with sliced sweet
oranges or candied peel.

Citrus × aurantium
BITTER ORANGE

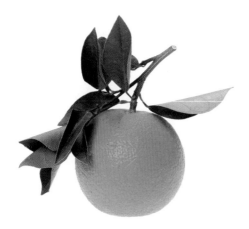

A feel-good fruit, bitter or sour orange is said to calm frazzled nerves, and science has confirmed its ability to calm, relax, and act as a mild sedative.

ABOUT THE PLANT: A small tree from Asia, East Africa, Arabia, and Syria, it's cultivated in the Mediterranean, the southern United States, South Africa, Australia, and the Caribbean to produce the fruit used in marmalade. Its bitterness distinguishes it from close relatives bergamot and sweet orange. It has long, leathery green leaves, and its sweet-fragranced, yellowish-white flowers make one of the most beautifully scented essential oils.

HISTORY AND FOLKLORE: A universal calming balm, bitter orange has been traditionally used in Chinese, Japanese, Ayurvedic, South American and Western herbal medicine for anxiety, as a sedative for minor insomnia, in epilepsy, and as a tonic to strengthen the nervous systems of adults and children. Basque people have historically used its leaves for insomnia and palpitations. The oils are used in perfumery, and the oil and peel in flavoring such as orange liqueurs. Bitter orange is added to supplements to increase appetite and help weight loss.

WHAT SCIENTISTS SAY

In humans: Bitter orange flower extracts and inhalation of its beautifully scented essential oil (neroli) have been shown in initial clinical trials to significantly reduce anxiety. Neroli essential oil also clinically reduces blood pressure and anxiety and improves sleep in coronary patients when inhaled with lavender and Roman chamomile. It reduces blood pressure and cortisol levels in hypertension when inhaled with other essential oils. Bitter orange extract has also been shown to alleviate anxiety and pain in labor. Commercial extracts, not the essential oil, increased blood pressure in some but not all trials. In a controlled trial, sweet orange (*Citrus × sinensis*) improved cognitive function in older people.

In the lab: Studies show bitter orange is sedative, reduces spasms, and is anticonvulsant via the brain's calming (GABA) signal and also by blocking the brain's stimulatory (glutamate) signal. It also has antidepressant effects via the mood-boosting (serotonin) neurotransmitter, and the flower extract, peel, and seeds are the all-important neuroprotective with antioxidant and anti-inflammatory properties.

KEY INGREDIENTS: Contains naringin (also in bergamot and grapefruit), a flavonoid studied for use in anxiety, epilepsy, for memory, and as a neuroprotective. Contains the sedative ingredient hesperidin which is also in passionflower and valerian. Fruit and flower contain alkaloids that have adrenergic (weight loss) effects. Essential oils from bitter orange don't contain the alkaloids. Three essential oils are produced from different parts of this plant—"bitter orange" (from peel), "neroli" (from flowers), and "petitgrain" (from leaves and wood, which can sometimes confusingly include essential oils from other plants). Neroli contains linalool (the constituent in lavender and other calming plants) and the peel oil differs in being almost identical to sweet orange.

HOW TO TAKE IT: Best for calming is neroli essential oil used in aromatherapy. Fresh flower tea or peel decoction, tincture, or extracts are also commonly used. Cook with peel syrup, try bitter orange caramelized potatoes, or simply enjoy marmalade on toast.

SAFETY: At medicinal doses of the extract, not in heart conditions, high blood pressure, glaucoma, ischemic colitis, or with monoamine oxidase inhibitors for depression. Juice may increase bioavailability of drugs, similar to grapefruit. Bitter orange peel (not neroli flower) oil is moderately phototoxic (do not use above 1 percent on skin application). The extract can increase heart rate; take care when using supplements where active ingredients may be increased and where caffeine increases this effect.

Bitter orange extract is regulated by the US Food and Drug Administration on account of its overuse in weight loss supplements. The peel, oil, and extracts are generally recognized as safe (GRAS) as a direct additive to food.

Cramp bark

Viburnum opulus (cramp bark or guelder rose) is a large deciduous shrub used in Native American medicine for anxiety. A member of the honeysuckle family and native to Africa, Asia, and Europe, it is widespread on waysides there and has naturalized in much of North America. Substantial traditional evidence from around the world underlines its ability to calm both mind (antianxiety) and body (relaxant, antispasmodic, hypotensive). Medical herbalists recommend 10 g dried bark to be simmered in 375 ml water and 10 ml to be drunk 3 times daily. Canadians use the berries as a cranberry substitute in a savory jelly. Science on cramp bark has yet to emerge.

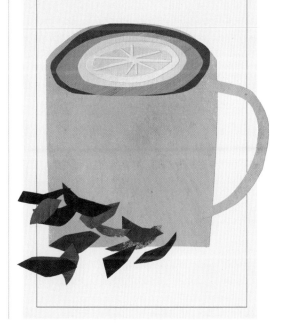

Yoga on the chamomile lawn

Yoga is the classic practice proven to calm the mind and relax the body. Performing yoga on a chamomile lawn doubles the benefit—your deep breaths and stretches will relax muscles and relieve anxiety and you will also be inhaling the calming chamomile aromatic chemicals such as alpha-pinene that reach your brain to increase calming brain signals (GABA).

The nonflowering Roman chamomile (*Chamaemelum nobile*) makes the best lawn and is really easy to grow. Just cordon off some of your lawn and plant runners on it, or make a chamomile "yoga mat" by growing plants on a slightly raised bed—lovely just to lie on. A lawn will thrive under the pressure of your footfall. As Shakespeare's Falstaff said of chamomile, "The more it is trodden on the faster it grows," so walking on it will be of mutual benefit for both you and the plants.

If you don't have a chamomile lawn, any lawn will do—just sprinkle 5 to 10 drops of Roman chamomile oil on your yoga mat. The volatiles will soon reach your brain to give the same benefits as the lawn.

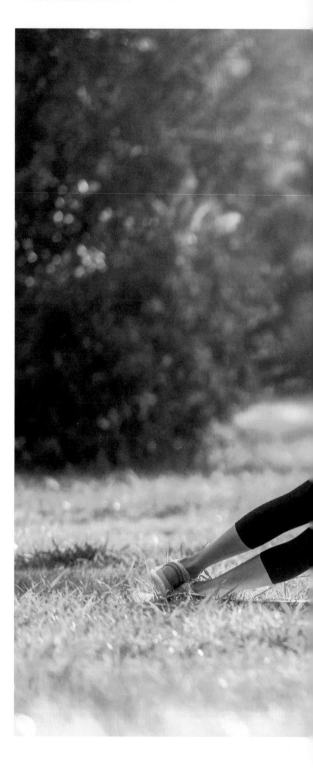

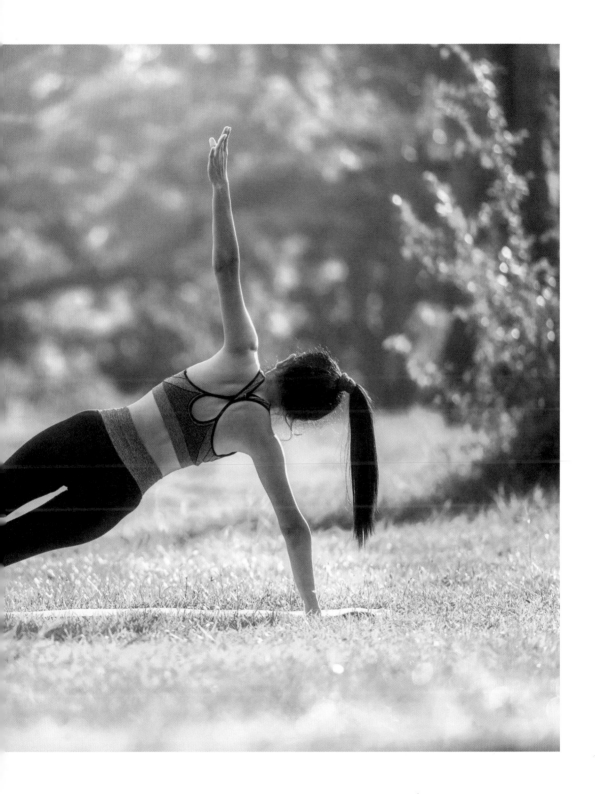

Bergamot banana bread

Makes 1 loaf

FOR THE BREAD:

2 cups (250 g) all-purpose flour

½ cup (125 g) light brown sugar

Pinch of salt

1 teaspoon baking powder

3 medium-ripe bananas, peeled

1 tablespoon grated bergamot
   orange zest

3½ tablespoons (50 g) butter,
   melted

2 eggs, beaten

FOR THE TOPPING:

5 drops bergamot orange
   essential oil

¼ cup (60 ml) lemon curd

¾ cup (85 g) walnut halves

1 banana, sliced

Calming bergamot teamed with mood-boosting banana makes a satisfyingly cake-like bread.

❶ Preheat the oven to 375°F (190°C) and line the base and sides of an 8 by 4-inch (20 by 10 cm) loaf pan with parchment paper.

❷ Sift the dry ingredients into a bowl and mix well.

❸ Place the bananas in a bowl and mash with a fork, then add the grated zest, melted butter, and beaten eggs.

❹ Fold the wet ingredients into the dry ingredients and loosely combine.

❺ Pour into the prepared loaf tin and bake for 45 minutes or until a skewer comes out clean.

❻ Remove from the oven, leave to cool in the tin then transfer to a wire rack.

❼ For the icing, add the bergamot oil to the lemon curd and spread a thin layer to the top of the loaf. Decorate with walnut halves and pieces of sliced banana.

Citrus × bergamia syn. *Citrus limon*

BERGAMOT

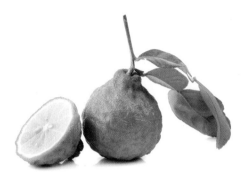

A feel-good fruit with relaxing, anxiety-relieving ingredients. Great as a juice or tea, there is growing science to verify its ability to calm. Also contains the super-brain flavonoid naringin.

ABOUT THE PLANT: An aromatic perennial, this hybrid of bitter orange and lemon originated in tropical Asia and grows wild and is cultivated in southern Italy. It is a small evergreen tree with pointed dark green leaves and fragrant star-shaped white flowers. The small pear-shaped, green- to yellow-skinned fruit is picked unripe for its juice and aromatic peel and has a fresh, sweet, floral scent. The scent and flavor of wild bergamot (*Monarda fistulosa*) is similar to *Citrus × bergamia* (both essential oils contain pinene and terpinene) and confusingly this plant is also called bergamot.

HISTORY AND FOLKLORE: Thought to have been brought by Columbus from the Canary Islands to Berga in Spain, it made its way to Italy, and the uplifting yet relaxing *Citrus × bergamia* was a key remedy in Italian folk medicine and from the sixteenth century in European herbals. Bergamot comes from the Italian word *bergamotto* of Turkish origin (*beg-armudi* or *beg armut*), meaning prince of pears. It was a key ingredient of classic eau-de-cologne in Napoleonic times and is still used in perfumery and foodstuffs, adding the distinct aroma to Earl Grey tea. The essential oil is sometimes used in suntan oils.

WHAT SCIENTISTS SAY

In humans: A small number of clinical studies confirm that bergamot relaxes when used with other calming plants. In pilot studies it lowers pulse rate and blood pressure when given transdermally (massaged into skin) with lavender, and it also relaxes when inhaled while listening to music. It reduces depression and pain in cancer patients on hand massage with lavender and frankincense. Inhaled (with lavender and ylang-ylang) it lowers blood pressure, pulse, and cortisol, and subjective stress and anxiety in hypertension.

In the lab: It boosts the calming (GABA) signal and lowers anxiety and the stress (corticosterone) response. It has pain-relieving effects (via cannabinoid and opioid signals), changing the nerve cells' adaptability to pain. It's also anti-inflammatory and antioxidant, which are key to maintaining brain health.

KEY INGREDIENTS: Bergamot oil is distinct from other citrus oils. Expressed from the fruit peel, its main ingredients are limonene and the calming linalool and linalyl acetate. It also contains pinene. Bergapten is anti-inflammatory and caryophyllene is pain relieving. The peel and juice contain flavonoids such as neoeriocitrin and the brain-boosting naringin.

HOW TO TAKE IT: Fresh naringin-containing bergamot juice and extracts, or fresh or dried leaves and flowers as a tea, 4 to 6 g per 240 ml water 3 times daily. Use in aromatherapy and less than 0.4% of final product for massage. Also use the fruit with or instead of bitter oranges to make marmalade.

SAFETY: This particular essential oil on the skin may be phototoxic (so only use up to 0.4%) due to presence of bergapten and bergamottin (furanocoumarins)—to avoid this potential risk, you can buy bergapten-free oil.

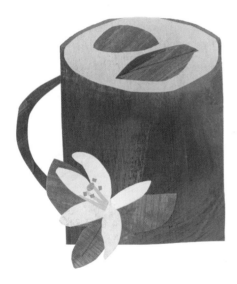

Leonurus cardiaca
MOTHERWORT

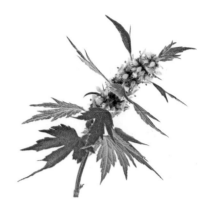

Motherwort has been used to treat anxiety and nervous heart conditions in Europe since the sixteenth century, and now science can show how it works.

ABOUT THE PLANT: A tall perennial widely found growing on the waysides of temperate Europe, Asia, and North America. Grows up to 5 feet (1.5 m) with palm-shaped, deep-toothed dark leaves and two-lipped white to pink flowers that blossom in clusters. Looks like mugwort when not flowering. Closely related medicinally to *Leonurus japonicus*, used for women's health in Asia, and South African *Leonotis leonurus* (known as wild cannabis, which has mind-altering effects). It has a pungent odor and a bitter taste. Aerial parts harvested on flowering.

HISTORY AND FOLKLORE: Called lion's tail (Greek: *Leon oura*) due to prickly calyx teeth around its flowers. The English herbalist Culpeper said, "There is no better herb to drive away melancholy vapours from the heart." The species name *cardiaca* suggests its longstanding use in herbal medicine for nervousness, palpitations, and as a heart tonic, improving heart function and blood circulation. Italian doctor and herbalist Mattioli described it as "useful for palpitations and a pounding heart, to strengthen it and make the mind cheerful." Used in Chinese and Japanese medicine for cardiovascular and gynecological disorders and menopause.

WHAT SCIENTISTS SAY

In humans: Initial human pilot trials confirm its use for anxiety and as a hypotensive. An oil extract reduced symptoms of anxiety and depression in hypertensive patients and an extract improved the emotional state in anxious young people.

In the lab: Studies confirm it is calming (via the GABA signal) and has pain-relieving, anti-inflammatory, and antioxidant effects. Affects the circulatory system (anticoagulant), protects the heart, and has neuroprotective effects in lab tests.

KEY INGREDIENTS: Alkaloids such as leonurine, which has a mild psychoactive effect and acts on calming (GABA) pathways, and stachydrine, which shows hypotensive and neuroprotective effects in the lab. Also contains brain-boosting flavonoids such as hyperoside, lavandulifolioside, phenolic acids, and tannins.

HOW TO TAKE IT: A tea of dried (4 to 6 g) or fresh (6 to 12 g) aerial parts per 240 ml water 3 times per day. Tincture, capsules, and tablets (often with other calming plants) are also used. Aerial parts are fried fresh or added to soups in Asia.

SAFETY: Do not use during pregnancy or heavy menstruation.

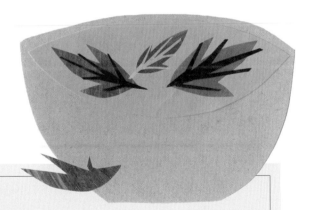

Motherwort

This plant is a great summer addition to savory Asian dishes. Fry fresh flowers and shoots with sesame oil and ginger and eat as is or add to chicken or fish soup.

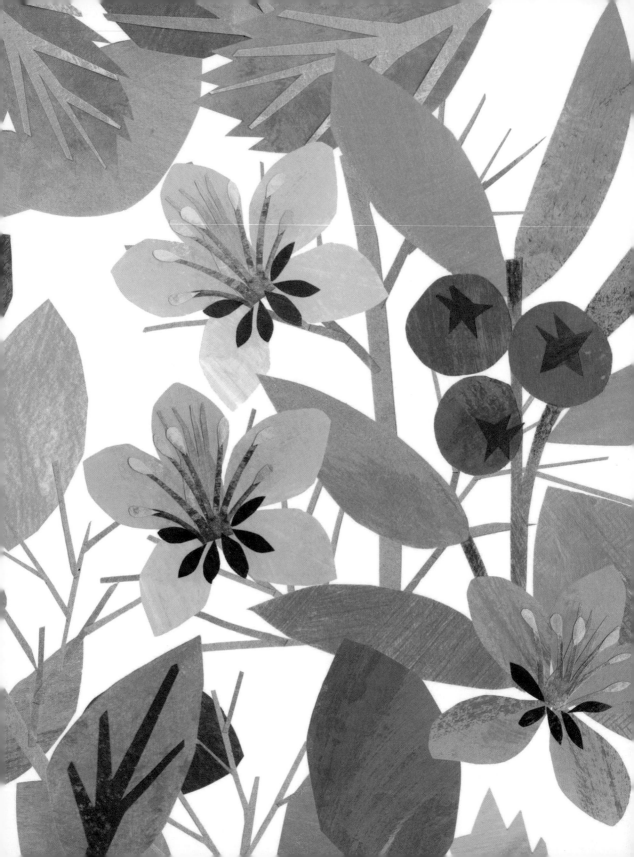

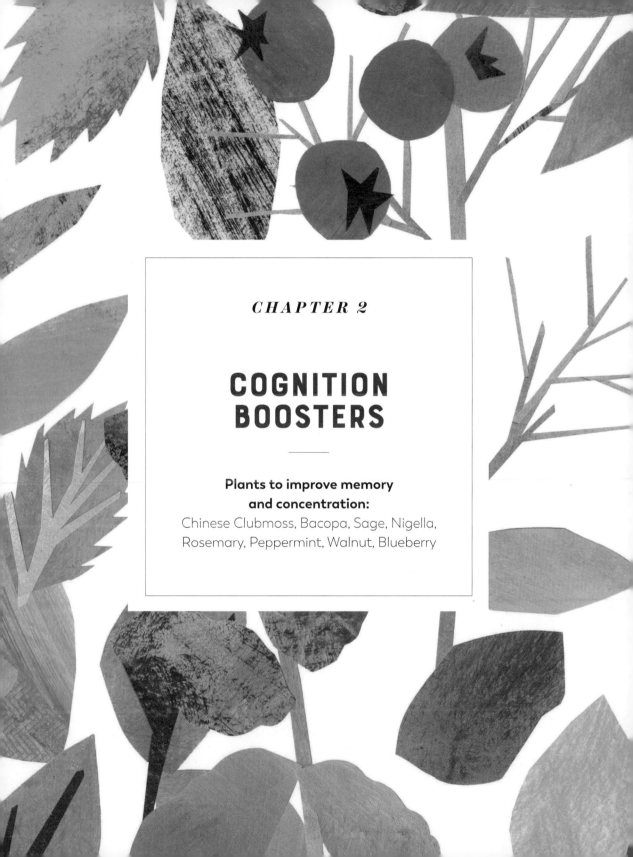

CHAPTER 2

COGNITION BOOSTERS

**Plants to improve memory
and concentration:**
Chinese Clubmoss, Bacopa, Sage, Nigella,
Rosemary, Peppermint, Walnut, Blueberry

At various times in our lives we may look for ways to improve our concentration, attention, comprehension, and memory. Students use cognition-enhancing drugs such as modafinil and metamphetamine so they can stay awake to study longer. Elderly people with dementia are given drugs such as galantamine from the snowdrop, which helps to relieve memory loss. But beyond these particular stress points many people reaching middle age begin to notice they don't remember events and facts quite as well as they used to and this is the time to start using plants to boost memory and protect the brain.

Below: *Narcissus pseudonarcissus* (daffodil) and *Galanthus nivalis* (snowdrop) **opposite** are both sources of galantamine, which is used to treat dementia.

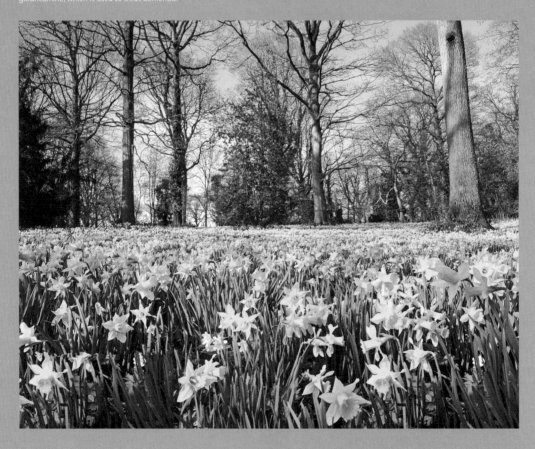

YOUR BRAIN ON PLANTS

Most of us over 60 will experience some sort of memory decline, with changes in cognitive function and brain structure. Retaining information and experience is a vital part of our identity and conscious awareness, and there are plants that science has shown can help in this. It was the science of "cognitive plants" that took our research on a new road and led to the creation of the Dilston Physic Garden in the wilds of Northumberland.

A BLOOMING AREA FOR DISCOVERY

It has been twenty years since we first turned our attention to plants as promising aids in the treatment of memory loss and dementia. The common garden herb sage, best known for adding flavor to the stuffing when cooking poultry, surprised us. We included it in lab tests because of its long-standing reputation in old herbals for helping memory. In 1597, English herbalist John Gerard wrote in *The Herball or Generall Historie of Plantes* that sage was "singularly good for the head and brain. It quickeneth the sense and memory." Our research more than 400 years later shows that sage (*Salvia officinalis* and *S. lavandulaefolia*) and other well-known household herbs such as lemon balm (*Melissa officinalis*) work on brain memory signals to improve memory, tested in the lab and tested in trials against placebo. Gerard was right.

Testing plants for use in cognition is now a thriving research area around the world. Since the early days of our research, the number of papers published on plants implicated in memory improvement has risen from under 20 to over 200 a year. The incentives are great, for example the need for new therapies for Alzheimer's disease, which affects so many in old age. And expectations are realistic: two of today's treatments are based on drugs that

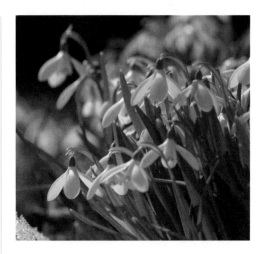

come from plants. A drawback is that the plants providing these drugs (galantamine from snowdrops or daffodils and rivastigmine from the calabar bean) are highly toxic, which means side effects such as nausea are a problem. For this chapter, we have picked out eight botanical brain balms for memory and concentration that are not toxic, and you can be confident that their therapeutic effect is backed by hundreds of years of use, along with clear evidence from the lab and from tests on humans.

Take a walk in the wild

A Stanford University study found that 30 participants who walked through green areas of campus for 50 minutes had benefits in cognition, such as working memory, and afterwards were more attentive and happier, with less anxiety and rumination, compared to the 30 strolling near heavy urban traffic.

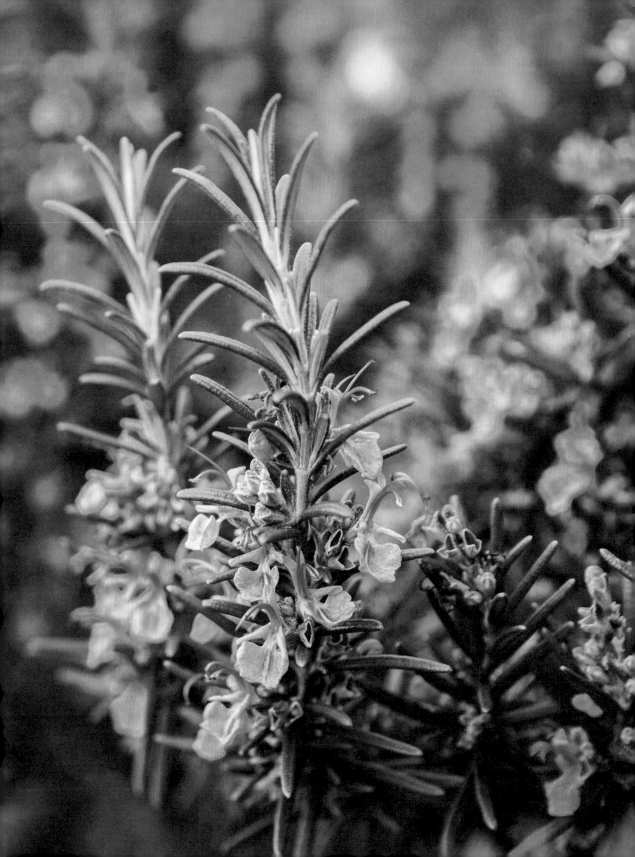

THE SCIENCE OF BOOSTING BALMS

Our cognition boosters involve the brain's memory and attention signal—acetylcholine. Vital to learning and awareness, this stimulatory neurotransmitter helps us to maintain attention, think clearly, and remember. In Alzheimer's, this memory signal (cholinergic) system is impaired. Acetylcholine is the most studied brain signal for memory and dementia, and it is significant that it decreases as we age. Plants for cognition contain ingredients that boost and hold this memory signal in the brain. They prevent it from being broken down by an enzyme and thereby enhance its effect. Other brain signals (such as the glutamate and its NMDA [N-methyl-D-asparate] receptor) are also involved in memory. Also key to maintaining brain health and cognition are anti-inflammatory and antioxidant plant ingredients that many plants manufacture for their own survival. Some plants, including sage and rosemary, are rich sources of these.

Opposite: Lab studies show that *Rosmarinus officinalis* (rosemary) enhances blood capillary flow, which may account for beneficial effects that range from brain function to hair growth.

COGNITIVE BOTANICAL CHOICES

Our portfolio of eight science-backed cognitive plants includes the now-famous brain-boosting sage, well-known household herbs such as peppermint and rosemary, the exotic bacopa (an Ayurvedic medicine), clubmoss, and nigella, and the common edibles walnut and blueberry. The boosting balms are listed in order of the strongest to the least scientific evidence as cognitive enhancers.

Many plants in other chapters have an impact on memory, and clinical trials show positive effects on memory in humans. These include ashwagandha, gotu kola, jujube, turmeric, lemon balm, citrus fruits, and the most intensively investigated ginkgo. In laboratories throughout the world a huge number of plants are undergoing scientific exploration for memory, and there are many more that are supported by traditional use but have no science behind them yet.

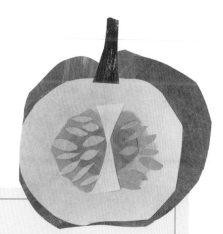

Don't forget your fruit and veg

They're full of carotenoids such as lutein and polyphenols like resveratrol, which are also present in many plants in this book. These compounds are correlated with better cognitive ability in humans studies and are neuroprotective in the lab.

COGNITIVE PLANTS WITH EXPLORATORY HUMAN STUDIES

Exploratory tests in humans show that saffron crocus (*Crocus sativus*), native to southern Europe and Asia, improves memory in healthy adults and in people with Alzheimer's. Lab tests have shown its yellow ingredient, crocin, is able to improve memory and be neuroprotective and antioxidant. Kesum (*Persicaria maculosa*) is used for flavoring in Malaysia, and in a study involving 35 middle-aged women has also improved attention, short-term memory, IQ, and mood. The flavonoid-rich Concord grape (*Vitis labrusca* cultivar) improved memory in preteen children and in older adults—as did the crop plant oat (*Avena sativa*). Roseroot (*Rhodiola rosea* syn. *Sedum roseum*) is shown in several human studies to aid concentration and memory, relieve fatigue and stress, and to be neuroprotective and stimulatory in lab work, too. Ginger (*Zingiber officinale*) has enhanced memory in 60 middle-aged women against a placebo, and in the lab it improves memory, promotes brain cell growth, and decreases brain inflammation.

COGNITIVE PLANTS WITH POSITIVE LAB TESTS

The following plants have been shown to increase the memory signal acetylcholine and improve memory in the lab: mucuracaá (*Petiveria alliacea*), pomegranate (*Punica granatum*), eastern bamboo (*Phyllostachys*), jujube (*Ziziphus jujube* var. *spinosa*), white birch (*Betula platyphylla*), peppermint-scented holy basil or tulsi (*Ocimum tenuiflorum*), asparagus (*Asparagus* spp.), coriander (*Coriandrum sativum*) and cumin (*Cuminum cyminum*). The ingredient rhein in Chinese native rhubarb (*Rheum* spp.), imperatorin in the statuesque angelica (*Angelica archangelica*) and compounds in basket fern (*Drynaria* spp.) have been shown to improve memory in lab tests, too. Fumitory (*Fumaria officinalis* and other species), which used to be smoked for "disorders of the head," also increases the memory signal acetylcholine and affects other memory signals, too.

TRADITIONAL BOOSTING BALMS YET TO BE TESTED BY SCIENCE

Many more plants will come to be recognized by science for improving memory. These include the Scottish native cowslip (*Primula veris* syn. *P. officinalis*), famous for its narcotic juice and used in cowslip wine. In old herbals, cowslip was said to be good for memory and "paines in the head." And wood betony (*Betonica officinalis* syn. *Stachys betonica*), found in the woodlands of Europe, Asia, and North Africa, has acquired masses of historical traditional evidence that shows it can improve blood flow to the brain as well as boost memory and concentration.

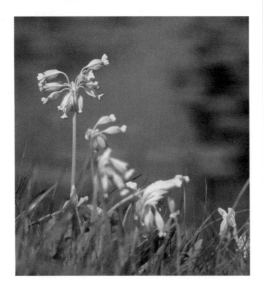

Left: *Primula veris* (cowslip) is often listed as a plant to improve memory in traditional herbals.
Opposite: *Phyllostachys* spp. (bamboo) has been shown to improve memory in lab tests.

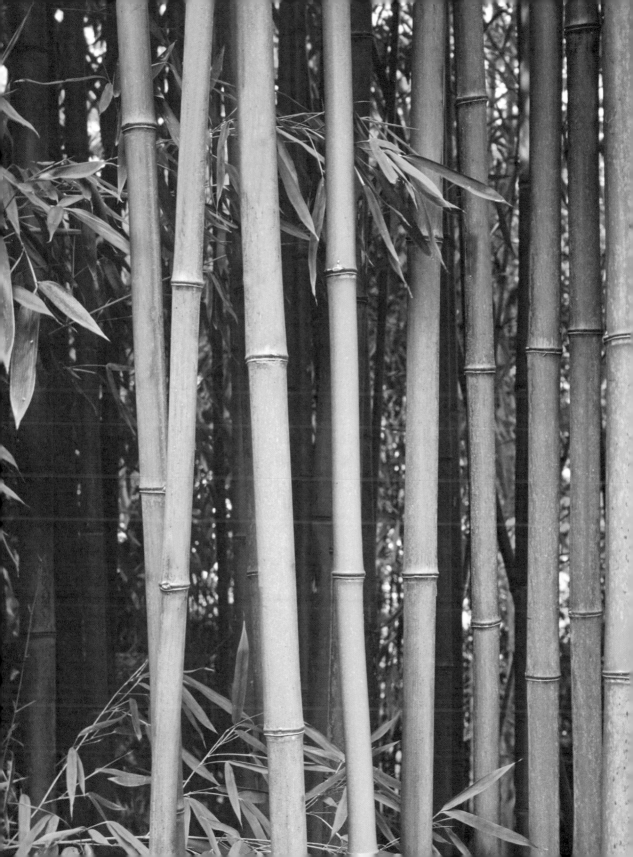

Huperzia serrata syn. *Lycopodium serratum*

CHINESE CLUBMOSS

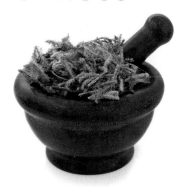

This traditional Chinese medicine for memory took the world by storm fifty years ago. Clinical studies show its ingredient huperzine is an effective cognitive enhancer that boosts learning, memory, and mood in students and people with Alzheimer's, and it is safe to take.

ABOUT THE PLANT: Also known by the common names toothed or fir clubmoss, this genus is one of the oldest plants on the planet, for it grew 390 million years ago when tree forms of clubmoss reached heights of 100 feet (30 m). Now growing to about 12 inches (30 cm), the slow-growing, evergreen clubmoss looks very much like a large moss with branching green stems and simple needle-like leaf structures called microphylls. In China it is becoming endangered but can still be found largely in rock crevices and damp forests along the Changjiang River area, and it also grows in tropical and subtropical forests of Australia and India. Also known as ground pine or creeping cedar, it is epiphytic, slow-growing, and propagated mainly by spores. It does not produce flowers.

HISTORY AND FOLKLORE: This ancient Chinese plant remedy dating back to 600 to 900 AD, brewed as a tea, Qian Ceng Ta, has been used to treat various mental disorders, fever, and inflammation. Chinese medicine practitioners noticed that people who drank the tea found their memories improved. Spores from the related species wolf's claw clubmoss (*Lycopodium clavatum*, common throughout the world), ignite when thrown into flame. Once thought to be magic, this practice provided the flash in early photography.

WHAT SCIENTISTS SAY

In humans: Chinese clubmoss was discovered to be a brain booster in China in the 1970s when people using it had nausea and dizziness (a sign of overstimulus of memory signals). Numerous clinical studies in China show its active ingredient huperzine is an effective cognitive enhancer. Controlled studies show beneficial effects in learning and memory in students, in a meta-analysis for Alzheimer's, in vascular and multi-infarct dementia, and in cocaine use disorder, as well as beneficial effects in initial studies of brain trauma, schizophrenia, and benign senescent forgetfulness. Huperzine was approved to treat Alzheimer's in the 1990s and improves memory, cognition, mood, and behavioral function.

In the lab: Huperzine works by potently boosting the memory signal acetylcholine, and also affects another memory signal, glutamate, improving learning and memory in various (including cognitively impaired) lab models. Huperzine also has strong neuroprotective effects, lowering inflammation, affecting gene expression and mitochondrial dysfunction in brain disorder models, and increasing neuronal growth.

KEY INGREDIENTS: The *Lycopodium* alkaloids huperzine A and B (and others such as carinatumin) boost the memory signal acetylcholine. Members of the genus *Phlegmariurus* in the same family contain more huperzine A than Huperzia species.

HOW TO TAKE IT: Commonly taken in capsules or powder form, and capsules of the active ingredient huperzine A on its own are also taken. Aerial parts can be taken as a tea or added to your morning smoothie. Not to be mistaken for *Lycopodium clavatum* (a related species that does not contain the active huperzine). Consult your health care practitioner as dose can vary with health, age, and weight.

SAFETY: Reported entirely safe in recommended dose. Do not exceed recommended dose to avoid side effects such as blurred vision, nausea, and vomiting. More studies are required, though huperzine A is reported to have high tolerance, with no serious adverse events. Do not take in pregnancy, hypertension, epilepsy, heart conditions (it can change the heart rate), or pulmonary disorders (it increases mucous).

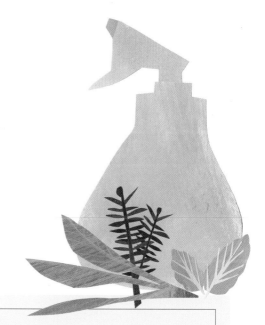

Sage, pine, and mint cleaning spray

Make up this everyday household cleaning spray using plants that have cleansing and brain-boosting properties. Add equal amounts of the pure essential oils of sage, pine, and mint to an alcohol base using 1 to 2 parts oil per 100 parts base (or adjust proportion to preferred scent). Shake and leave to disperse. Bottle in a dark container with spray attachment. Spray liberally over working surfaces in kitchen or your work desk to surround yourself in brain-boosting aromas. Most surfaces will not be damaged by the spray oils, which quickly evaporate, but always test a small area first. The spray can be stored for at least one year.

Pines for memory

Himalayan pine (*Pinus roxburghii*, named after William Roxburgh, the famous Scottish surgeon and botanist) improves memory in the lab, and the bark of Monterey pine (*P. radiata*) improves cognitive function in people with brain injury. In a study in Melbourne, Australia, *P. radiata* administered to forty-two males increased the speed of memory. The active ingredients of pine are thought to be flavonoids and superlipids (polyprenols), but pines also contain the chemical alpha-pinene, which is known to boost the memory signal acetylcholine in the brain.

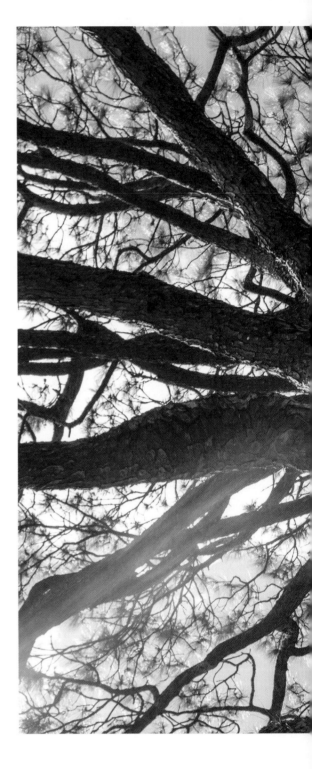

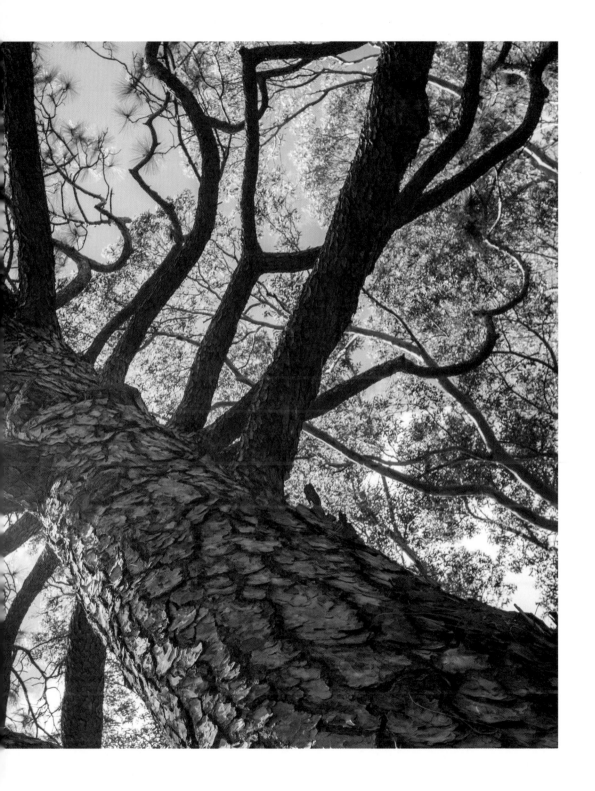

Bacopa monnieri

BACOPA

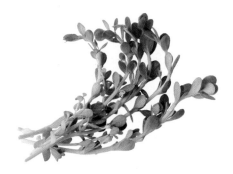

This succulent swamp plant used in Ayurvedic medicine is increasingly being recognized for its effects on memory as a result of scientific research. It has memory, antiaging, and brain health properties, and also has positive results for attention-deficit-hyperactivity disorder (ADHD) in children.

ABOUT THE PLANT: This perennial creeping plant, known as water hyssop, is found in marshy subtropical regions in India and Australia. Forming dense mats in mangrove swamp edges, it has oblong fleshy leaves with small nonaromatic white or pale blue flowers. Readily obtained from garden centers, various species of bacopa are used as pond plants for aeration.

HISTORY AND FOLKLORE: With other names such as herb of grace and brahmi after the Hindu god of creation, this plant was originally described in the sixth century. Ayurvedic texts extol its use for memory, calming, and nervous system disorders. Not yet part of Western herbal medical texts or teachings, bacopa is used in India as a tonic for neurological conditions, as well as for other non-brain disorders. The expressed juice is sometimes mixed with oil and applied for arthritic pain.

WHAT SCIENTISTS SAY: Subject to hundreds of studies in Australia and India.

In humans: Bacopa improves cognition, attention, and memory in healthy people in controlled trials and in those who have mild cognitive impairment. It also safely reduces symptoms of ADHD in children, reduces depression, anxiety, and heart rate in the elderly, and improves mood and performance in multitask stress activities in controlled studies.

In the lab: Bacopa increases the memory signal acetylcholine and affects the excitatory signal (glutamate) and the mood and reward signals (serotonin and dopamine). It's also neuroprotective, promotes growth of new nerve cells, and increases blood flow to the brain. With key brain-boosting, anti-inflammatory, and antioxidant properties, it increases longevity in tests mimicking aging.

KEY INGREDIENTS: The best-characterized neuroactives are the triterpene saponins called bacosides. Also contains alkaloids (like brahmine).

HOW TO TAKE IT: Studies show fresh aerial parts (leaves and stems, up to 10 g daily) are best and can be made into pesto and dal. Dried and stored (for no longer than three months) they can be taken made into a paste, tincture, or tea. Also available as capsules and tablets. May take up to twelve weeks for cognitive effects, but anxiety-relieving effects are more immediate.

SAFETY: Advisable to take with food but not on a full stomach as it may cause indigestion. Caution in thyroid, antidepressant, and sedative medication.

Salvia officinalis and *S. lavandulaefolia*

SAGE

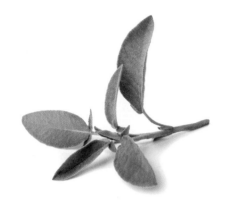

European sage (*Salvia officinalis*) is extolled for so many virtues relating to the well-being of mind and body that it's considered a "cure-all" in Europe. Our original research on sage, driven by its centuries-old reputation for enhancing memory, seeded the idea for Dilston Physic Garden.

ABOUT THE PLANT: These two sages are perennial woody shrubs with purple-blue flowers and silvery green leaves, more silver and narrower in Spanish sage, hence its Latin name—*lavandulaefolia*. They thrive on well-drained soil and in pots and are generally drought-tolerant and frost hardy. Leaves are harvested before flowering. Not to be confused with ornamental salvias, the hallucinogenic divine sage (*Salvia divinorum*), clary sage (*S. sclarea*) used in aromatherapy, or Chinese sage (*S. miltiorrhiza*), also active in the brain.

HISTORY AND FOLKLORE: Sage is valued globally as the key to a long life. The Chinese would exchange three cases of their tea for British sage tea. *Salvia* comes from the French *sauver*, meaning "to save," and this is reflected in old English sayings such as "why should a man die who has sage in his garden?" With a long-standing reputation for improving memory, sixteenth-century herbalists like Culpeper said it "is of excellent use to help the memory, warming and quickening the senses." Used by medical herbalists today as a stimulant and nerve tonic.

WHAT SCIENTISTS SAY: Studies here refer to *S. officinalis* or *S. lavandulaefolia* and include essential oil, alcohol, or water extracts.

In humans: In controlled trials sage enhances memory and alertness in healthy young and older people. It also improves attention in the elderly and counters cognitive impairment, as well as improving behavioral measures in Alzheimer's. Also improves mood measured by calmness and contentedness in volunteers. Lowers sore throat pain and has positive effects on blood lipid and antioxidant profile in controlled trials. In a pilot trial conducted at Dilston Physic Garden, with a health center and medical herbalist, taken with lemon balm and rosemary, sage improved the ability to recall a list of words by over 50 percent in under-63-year-olds.

In the lab: Improves memory in many lab models and protects against neuronal injury. Boosts the memory and awareness signal (acetylcholine) by blocking enzymes that break it down—monoterpenes, diterpenes and polyphenols like rosmarinic acid all do this. While thujone impairs memory in a lab model by inhibiting memory signals (via nicotinic receptor), camphor and borneol boost them. Different monoterpenes, diterpenes, and flavones also act on calming signals—and on two different parts of the calming GABA brain molecule.

Take a green break at work

The more you exercise the less risk you have of cognitive decline. During exercise, blood flow to specific parts of the brain, such as those involved in memory, increases by 200 percent. If possible, go to your nearest park or garden to exercise in the fresh air. Being in a green space has been shown to increase your working memory and reduce your cortisol levels. If you can't get out into the fresh air when doing exercise, try using sage, rosemary, or peppermint essential oil (a few drops on your shirt or workout mat) to improve cognition.

Regular repeated exercise triggers various changes in brain tissue, such as the growth of new cells and transmitters, and the production of brain-saving antioxidants. On top of this, the coordination required for movements such as doing simple star jumps stimulates cognitive function when practiced regularly. For those inclined toward more gentle forms of exercise there's evidence that stretching and strength training are also beneficial to boosting the brain. So try outdoor tai chi, yoga, tae kwon do, karate, ballet, Zumba— whatever coordinated exercise appeals to you.

KEY INGREDIENTS: Essential oil of *Salvia officinalis* contains cineole, camphor, thujone, borneol, and caryophyllene oxide. *S.lavandulaefolia* contains only trace amounts of thujone and is higher in cineole, pinenes, and camphor. Both species contain key neuroprotective and inflammation- and oxidation-reducing compounds from polyphenols like salvigenin and rosmarinic acid, to flavonoids like hispidulin, apigenin, and luteolin and various monoterpenes.

HOW TO TAKE IT: Teas from fresh (20 g) or dried (4 to 6 g) leaves per 240 ml water 3 times daily are particularly good with honey. Capsules, tablets, tinctures, sprays (water extracts for throat infections), and culinary preparations are also used—such as in the classic poultry stuffing or fried on its own, but effective medicinal doses may not be reached without regular consumption.

SAFETY: Safe at recommended dose and without side effects for most people. Thujone (in *Salvia officinalis*) means it's not suitable for children, pregnant women, or those with epilepsy. Both species contain camphor. Caution in raised blood pressure and in diabetes medication as *S.officinalis* clinically lowers blood sugar, and with hormone-sensitive conditions since sage is estrogenic.

Nigella sativa

NIGELLA

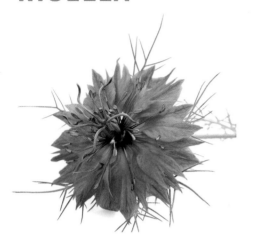

A medicinal plant favored in Arabic culture for hundreds of years for improving memory, nigella grows and flowers readily in colder climates (unlike Middle Eastern saffron, which has equally extensive mind and body benefits). Described as the Ayurvedic "miracle herb" it has an extraordinary range of health benefits, many of them backed by science.

ABOUT THE PLANT: This member of the buttercup family, which originates from southern Europe, North Africa, and Asia, is an annual that likes the sun. Growing to over 12 inches (30 cm) with an upright branching stem and finely divided leaves, it has delicate white or pale blue flowers. Its toothed black seeds form in seed heads similar to those of poppies and are gathered when ripe—when rubbed they have a peppery smell and taste similar to oregano.

HISTORY AND FOLKLORE: Also called black cumin, blessed seed, wild onion seed, kalonji, and *cheveux de venus* in France, the seeds were found in ancient Egyptian tombs. The prophet Mohammed described nigella's many healing powers, saying the only disease it can't cure is death. It's also referred to in the Bible (Isaiah) and was used by the first century AD Greek physician Dioscorides. It was placed in the London Pharmacopaeia in 1721. Used traditionally around the world for a wide variety of disorders from hypertension to headache, it's regarded as a high-ranking, evidence-based plant medicine.

WHAT SCIENTISTS SAY

In humans: In controlled clinical studies nigella enhanced cognition and verbal learning as well as mood, and relieved anxiety in healthy males. It also improved memory and attention in the elderly, reduced blood pressure and improved glycemic index (in controlled trials), and improved lipid profiles and immune function (in initial studies), all relevant to cognitive function. Nigella has been shown clinically to treat asthma, ear infections, dyspepsia, and arthritis, among other conditions, leading to its "miracle herb" status.

In the lab: Nigella is memory enhancing in various lab models. It increases the memory signals acetylcholine and glutamate, and shows antidepressive, antiepileptic, antipsychotic, and antioxidant effects. It is also neuroprotective against inflammation.

KEY INGREDIENTS: The bioactive thymoquinone from seeds, as well as alkaloids such as nigellicine and saponins. Essential oil contains carvacrol, thymol and the memory (and mood-boosting) alpha- and beta-pinenes.

HOW TO TAKE IT: Dried seeds 2 to 3 g daily though as it's a foodstuff it can be used liberally.

Dry-roast to bring out flavor and remove any bitterness and use in curries, salads, breads (maybe add honey), oils and in the spice mix panch phoron (delicious just added to boiling rice). Also available in capsules and as a seed powder or oil.

SAFETY: Not fully evaluated though all clinical trials report safety. Contact dermatitis and lowered blood pressure have been reported as side effects.

Rosmarinus officinalis

ROSEMARY

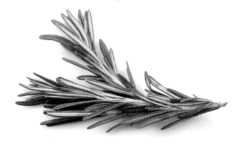

Renowned for being the herb for memory, both to enhance personal memory function and as a symbol of remembrance.

ABOUT THE PLANT: This Mediterranean native is a perennial woody plant that has uniquely fragrant, evergreen, needle-like leaves and pale pink or blue flowers. Preferring sun and well-drained soil, it thrives in pots and can reach 5 feet (1.5 m) in height. It is reasonably frost hardy and responds well to being pruned back regularly. Its tough, waxy leaves are insect resistant, and it may also protect nearby plants from pests.

HISTORY AND FOLKLORE: It is said that when the Virgin Mary spread her blue cloak over a white-blossomed rosemary bush while she was resting, the flowers turned blue. The shrub then became known as the "Rose of Mary." The ancient Greeks gave the herb to students to improve their memory, and students of Shakespeare's *Hamlet* will remember Ophelia saying "There's rosemary, that's for remembrance," which may reference the bard's neighbor, the sixteenth-century herbalist John Gerard. In the early seventeenth century, celebrated doctor of divinity Roger Hacket said in a sermon, "It overtoppeth all the flowers in the garden, boasting man's rule. It helpeth the brain, strengtheneth the memorie, and is very medicinable for the head." It is used in herbal medicine to improve mood, alleviate headaches and neuralgia, and treat palpitations; the essential oil is used as a stimulant.

WHAT SCIENTISTS SAY

In humans: Clinical studies show rosemary extract strengthens attention and memory in healthy students, adults, and the elderly. Used with lemon, orange, and lavender, it improves cognitive function in people with Alzheimer's. Research at Northumbria University in England has shown that the essential oil helps memory by 15 percent in the over-65s, and improves recall of events in the future (remembering to remember) by 70 percent. There are also clinical studies for its use in blood pressure control, anxiety, fatigue, and depression, and as an adjunct therapy to help with addictive drug withdrawal. Recently its long-held traditional use for promoting hair growth has also been proven.

In the lab: Studies show that rosemary enhances blood capillary flow, which may account for the beneficial effects from brain function to hair growth. It boosts the memory signal acetylcholine and acts on nicotine-like signals that increase attention. It's also anti-amyloid (reducing the brain protein plaques in Alzheimer's), neuroprotective, pain-relieving (serotonin and opioid receptors), acts on well-being signals (dopamine and serotonin), and is a key antioxidant and antidepressant (via serotonin signals). In fruit flies, it also extends life span.

KEY INGREDIENTS: Its distinguishing phenolic diterpenes such as carnosic and rosmarinic acids are important antioxidants and neuroprotective agents. Its volatile oil contains camphor, cineole, and borneol, which increase the memory signal acetylcholine in the lab and can reach the brain easily on inhalation.

HOW TO TAKE IT: Tea of leaves and flowers fresh (4 to 6 g) and dried (2 to 3 g) per 240 ml water 3 times daily. Tinctures, capsules, essential oil in aromatherapy also used. Rosemary is the ingredient in many culinary dishes—and makes an excellent infused oil for cooking.

SAFETY: Considered safe at the recommended dose, including during pregnancy. Not in epilepsy.

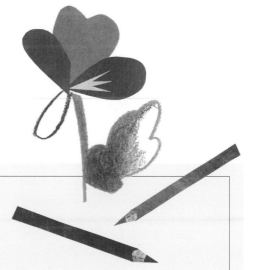

Remember a plant face

Hunt out a plant that you like the look of in the garden, park, or nearby garden center. Study it closely, noting its leaf and petal formation, how many sepals there are, what its pollen looks like, and the color and patterns of each part. Use a macro lens if you can—it's a whole new world! Then put it aside and sketch or paint it from your memory. Each time you do it, what you remember should improve a little.

   This is an effective way to enhance those memory signals; just as exercise keeps your muscles fit, so do brain exercises.

Breathe in the sage and rosemary

Breathe in to remember—but through your nose. A study in Chicago shows that people who see a series of faces remember them better, and two seconds faster, when inhaling through the nose, rather than when inhaling through the mouth or exhaling. Breathing stimulates and affects electrical activity in areas of the brain associated with memory, but that activity was shown to dissipate when the breath was taken through the mouth. Since studies show the aromas of sage, rosemary, and peppermint are brain boosters, breathing in their aroma through the nose is going to double the memory-stimulating effect.

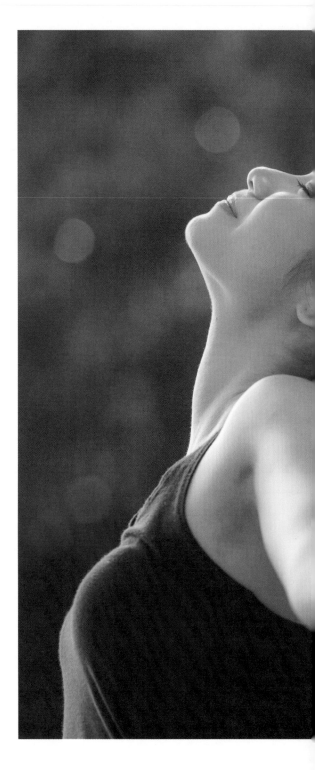

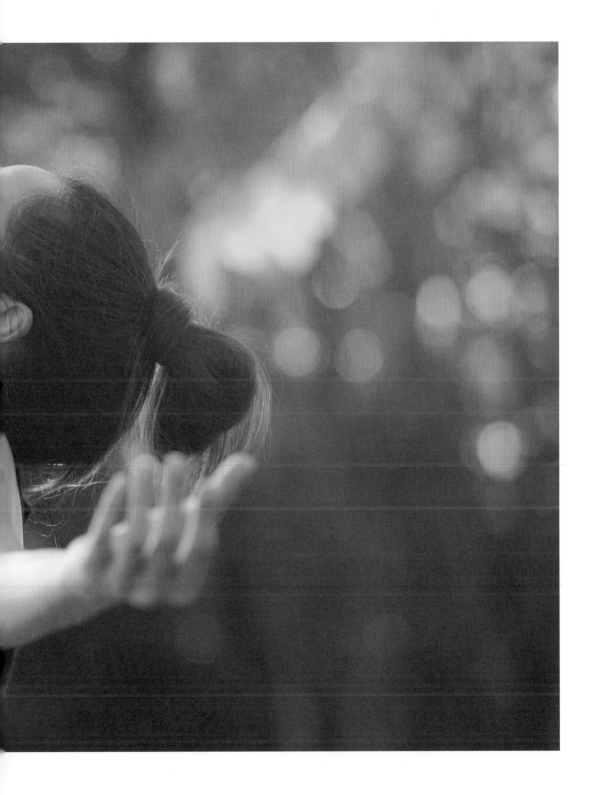

Mentha × piperita

PEPPERMINT

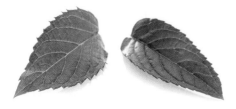

No other herb currently has such convincing evidence for combined body and mind use. With a robust reputation as an antispasmodic in modern mainstream medical practice, the science behind peppermint's long-held traditional use for boosting memory and alertness is only just being discovered.

ABOUT THE PLANT: This perennial plant is a cross between watermint and spearmint. It likes damp soils and uses wide-spreading rhizomes to increase; it is often grown in containers to check its invasive spread. It has dark green aromatic leaves with purple veins and pale pink-purple flowers. The medicinal properties of cultivars such as lime, lemon, and chocolate mint are unknown.

HISTORY AND FOLKLORE: Since the plant was originally described by Linnaeus in the eighteenth century, references in the old herbals do not apply to this species. The ancient Romans used other forms of mint in their feasting ceremonies, probably to aid digestion. Peppermint is a well-known ingredient of after-dinner chocolates, hard candies, and chewing gum and is the most popular single-ingredient herbal tea. Used by medical herbalists today as a stimulant for nervous disorders, "clearing" the mind, and the essential oil for alleviating mental fatigue and depression, improving

concentration, and reducing apathy. Also used to relieve pain (such as colic), nausea, and vomiting and to treat ulcerative colitis and Crohn's disease.

WHAT SCIENTISTS SAY

In humans: Studies show peppermint tea improves alertness, working memory, and long-term memory in 180 volunteers when compared to chamomile and hot water. Its aroma (essential oil) enhances memory and alertness in 144 volunteers compared to the aroma of ylang-ylang (which has the opposite effect). It also reduces perceived mental fatigue and prevents migraine progression. Unlike prescription drugs for cognition, peppermint is not associated with nausea—it's clinically antiemetic (postoperatively and in chemotherapy), and menthol from the oil is a safe and effective short-term treatment for irritable bowel in mainstream medicine.

In the lab: Mint species (such as *M. × piperata*, *M. aquatica* and *M. spicata*) and the flavonoid linarin found in wild mint (*M. arvensis*) and certain other mints boost the memory signal acetylcholine and are also stimulant, antioxidant, and neuroprotective. Menthol (present in various quantities in different mint species) affects memory and attention signals (via the stimulatory nicotinic receptor where acetylcholine works, and via glutamate) but also boosts the brain's calming (GABA) pathways. Menthol (and other chemical ingredients), peppermint, and other *Mentha* species (such as *M. spicata*) are also analgesic, relax gastro-intestinal spasms, modulate the immune system, and are antimicrobial and antiviral in the lab. Peppermint also activates skin receptors, leading to its classic cooling sensation.

KEY INGREDIENTS: Menthol, menthone, and linarin. The phenolics in the leaves include rosmarinic acid and several antioxidant flavonoids such as luteolin. Also contains small amounts of carvone that boost the stimulatory glutamate and inhibit the calming GABA signals.

HOW TO TAKE IT: Tea of leaves and flowering tops fresh (4 to 6 g) and dried (2 to 3 g) per 240 ml water 3 times daily. Tinctures, digestive spirits, capsules, and essential oil in aromatherapy also used. The essential oil can be taken orally for irritable bowel syndrome, where it is encapsulated. Also used in drinks and culinary dishes including confectionery.

SAFETY: Caution with gastric ulcers or reflux, gall bladder occlusions, hiatus hernia, or kidney stones. Do not allow children contact with the undiluted oil.

Humulus Lupulus

Have fun with Latin names

Many people find Latin plant names hard to remember, but they are essential to identifying the right plant. Make up ways of remembering Latin names of medicinal plants by inventing link words. Some botanical names are beautiful and by inventing fun link words remembering is a joy. For example, the wonderfully named *Atropa belladonna* (deadly nightshade), *Angelica archangelica* (angelica), *Humulus lupulus* (hops), *Hedera helix* (ivy), *Urtica urens* (nettle), *Salvia divinorum* (divine sage).

Juglans nigra, Juglans regia

WALNUT

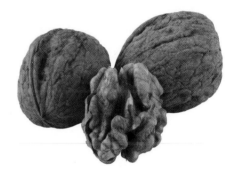

Walnuts are an example of the "doctrine of signatures" in which a food resembles one of its key health benefits, in this case the human brain.

ABOUT THE PLANT: *Juglans nigra* (black walnut) and *J. regia* (Eastern walnut) are deciduous trees that can live more than 200 years. They have pinnate leaves, and the black-skinned, hard-shelled nut (rounder in Eastern) is in two hemispheres.

HISTORY AND FOLKLORE: Also called Jupiter's nuts, from times when men supposedly lived on acorns and gods on walnuts. According to the sixteenth-century "doctrine of signatures" (where plants look like their medicinal use), the appearance of the two hemispheres of the walnut with its convoluted surface, so like the human brain, indicates its use for keeping the brain healthy. In the seventeenth century, English botanist William Cole said, "Laid upon the crown of the head, it comforts the brain and head mightily." While there is some clinical evidence for cognitive-enhancing effects, the capacity of the walnut to improve blood markers of hyperlipidemia, oxidative stress, and inflammation is likely to be as important for brain function.

WHAT SCIENTISTS SAY

In humans: The first human studies indicate that walnut consumption in adults (aged 20 to 90 years) increases all measures of cognition tested (such as reaction time and digit learning), and in students increases reasoning but not memory. Both nut and leaf lower blood triglycerides (more "good" and less "bad" cholesterol), reduce oxidative and inflammatory stress (markers of cardiac dysfunction in the blood), and reduce blood clotting risk, all relevant to maintaining brain function.

In the lab: Walnut improves memory, learning, and motor ability, enhances the brain's mood-boosting (serotonin) signals, lowers hypertension, and is neuroprotective against inflammation. Antioxidant effects are superior in English compared to black walnut (and many lab studies show anticancer effects).

KEY INGREDIENTS: Omega 3 (brain and heart health), diverse phenolics such as verulic and vanillic acids, and flavonoids, tannins, and quinones, notably the dark-staining juglone.

Go nuts for brain power. The David Geffen School of Medicine at UCLA looked at the effects of eating walnuts on cognitive function in the US between 1988 and 2002. Although the study relied on subjective reports of how many walnuts each person generally consumed, across 20-to-59-year-olds, eating more walnuts was significantly associated with better cognitive test scores. Though an epidemiological study that identifies trends and does not prove cause and effect, this study may say something for potential long-term preventative effects of plant chemicals on the brain.

HOW TO TAKE IT: Fresh, dried, or pickled nuts (up to 10 g daily—a "handful of walnuts") and fresh or dried leaves as a tea or tincture. Capsules also available—beware those for sale that are made from the walnut hull rather than the nuts themselves.

SAFETY: Due to the ingredient juglone, the outside capsule of the nut can stain and cause skin reactions—this was observed in horses bedded on walnut tree shavings. Discard nut if shell blackens. Overdosing is said to be a risk (liver and kidney), but there is no supporting scientific evidence.

Vaccinium corymbosum

BLUEBERRY

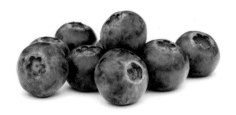

Blueberries are one of the most important contributions by Native Americans to world plant medicine. The berries are now among the top health foods in many countries and have been shown to improve memory in children and adults.

ABOUT THE PLANT: This perennial flowering shrub native to North America has white or pale pink, bell-shaped flowers and its famous purple berries have a powdery wax covering (bloom). Blueberries prefer acid soil and a sunny or part-shaded position. They will grow in pots but may only produce a few berries. The many related species include wild blueberry (*Vaccinium angustifolium*) and bilberry (*V. myrtillus*).

HISTORY AND FOLKLORE: Adopted internationally as a result of being so valued as a food and medicine by Native Americans. Not referred to in the old European herbals, which mention only the related bilberry (*Vaccinium myrtillus*). For several decades blueberries gained in popularity as a health food and are more recently appreciated for their brain-boosting capabilities.

WHAT SCIENTISTS SAY

In humans: In a trial in children aged 8 to 10 years a flavonoid-rich blueberry extract (freeze-dried) improved memory, and similarly in a pilot study so did blueberry juice. In older adults, trials show it stimulates venous function (blood flow back to heart), improves vascular function in men, and controls blood pressure (not supported by all reports). It also reduces oxidative stress, inflammation, and endothelial dysfunction in humans with cardiovascular risk factors, although single portions do not affect blood markers of oxidative stress. Also reduces insulin resistance in obese individuals (diabetes is linked to an increase in memory impairment) and enhances night vision.

In the lab: Blueberry improves learning and cognitive functions, promotes brain cell growth, reverses cognitive decline, and protects neurones from stress and cell membranes from inflammation, as well as being a significant antioxidant.

KEY INGREDIENTS: High concentrations of phenolic ingredients are key antioxidants. Anthocyanins and flavonoids such as quercetin and malvidin (also present in purple cabbage and beets) may be primarily responsible for health benefits, as well as for the blue-purple color. Some studies doubt anthocyanin bioavailability in the body.

HOW TO TAKE IT: Little can beat eating the fresh berries (60 to 100 g daily) but they can also be juiced, frozen, dried, or made into jellies, wine or spirits. Leaves (high in phenolics) can also be taken as a fresh tea or capsules, but don't contain all the brain-active ingredients in the fruit.

SAFETY: No evidence of drug interactions. Safe for children and pregnant women. Possible risk is amount of pesticides used in commercial products.

Fragrant blueberry and walnut muffins

Makes 12 muffins

8 tablespoons (1 stick/100 g) butter,
    at room temperature

1 cup (200 g) granulated sugar

1 teaspoon vanilla extract

2 large eggs

2 teaspoons baking powder

Pinch of salt

2 cups (240 g) all-purpose flour

1 cup (240 ml) milk

1 cup (200 g) blueberries

1 cup (100 g) walnuts, chopped

2 tablespoons chopped bacopa

1 tablespoon chopped rosemary

Stimulating rosemary and bacopa plus energizing fruit and nuts provide the perfect boost when you need to eat without losing focus.

❶ Heat the oven to 375°F (190°C) and place muffin cases in a 12-cup muffin pan.

❷ Cream the butter and sugar until pale and fluffy.

❸ Add the vanilla extract to the eggs and then slowly pour into the creamed butter and sugar, beating hard after each addition.

❹ Add the baking powder and a pinch of salt to the flour, then, using a spoon, alternately fold in the flour and the milk to the butter and sugar mixture.

❺ Fold in the blueberries, walnuts, bacopa, and rosemary and pour the batter into the prepared muffin pan.

❻ Bake for 15 to 20 minutes until golden brown. When ready they should spring back when lightly touched.

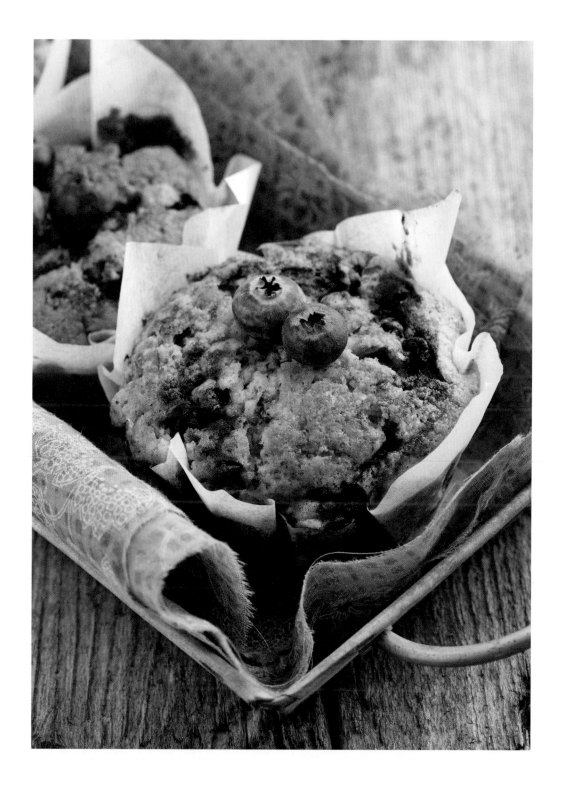

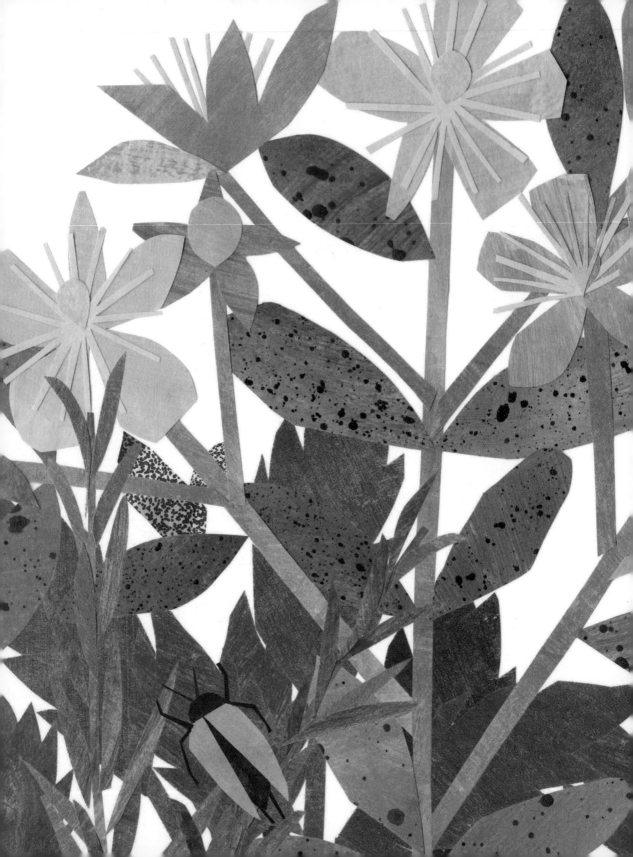

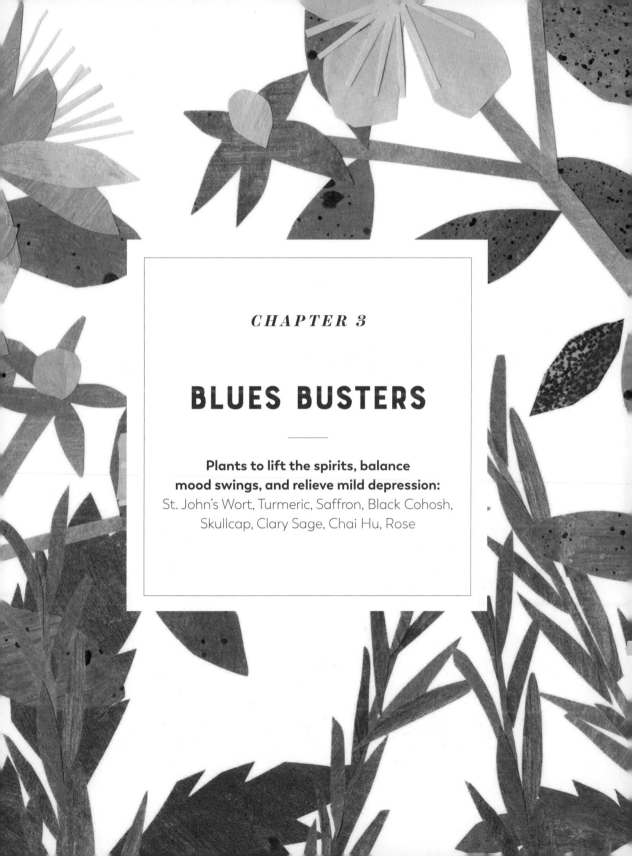

CHAPTER 3

BLUES BUSTERS

**Plants to lift the spirits, balance
mood swings, and relieve mild depression:**
St. John's Wort, Turmeric, Saffron, Black Cohosh,
Skullcap, Clary Sage, Chai Hu, Rose

The plants listed in this section are for lifting the mood, alleviating mild depression (severe depression should not be self-treated), and leveling out mood swings. The widely recognized antidepressive St. John's wort leads the way, but other traditional mood-boosting plants, successful in human studies, include turmeric and saffron from the Middle East and skullcap from Canada and the US.

Our list also includes, with lesser evidence, rose from the Middle East, chai hu from China, and, for restoring hormonal balance, particularly for women, there's black cohosh from the US and the less closely studied clary sage from Europe.

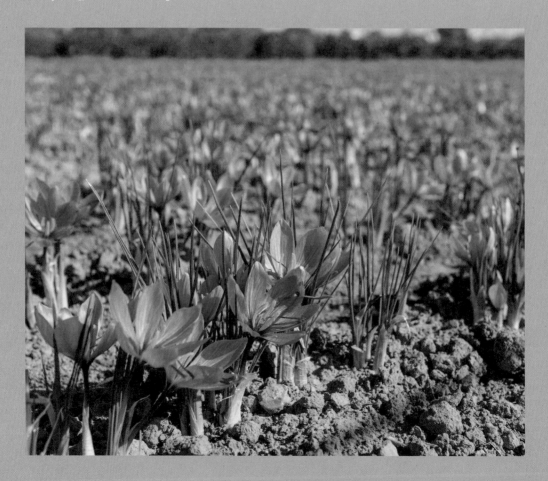

WHAT THE PLANTS NEED TO DO

A long-held notion surrounding depression is that it involves a response triggered by low brain serotonin levels and that drugs that restore this mood-boosting brain signal will also help to restore good mood. Consequently, common antidepressant drugs are those that are able to maintain high levels of serotonin in the space where nerve cells talk to each other (the synapse). These chemical drugs are collectively called SSRIs (selective serotonin reuptake inhibitors). They include fluoxetine (Prozac), sertraline, and paroxetine and are the most widely prescribed drugs today in the US, overtaking blood pressure drug prescription.

While some antidepressants act on serotonin, others act on noradrenaline and dopamine, for example the SNRIs (selective noradrenaline reuptake inhibitors), monoamine oxidase inhibitors, and TCAs (tricyclic antidepressants used more for severe depression).

Mild anxiety and depression are the most common of all mental health issues today, with one in five of us experiencing at least one episode of depression in our lifetime, so we need to be aware of different treatments and ask ourselves these questions. Do we fully understand what goes wrong in the brain-body-emotion axis during depression? Do SSRIs really work better than a placebo (an inert pill)? And are the side effects of SSRIs, which include nausea, dizziness and sexual problems, acceptable?

HOW WE BECAME INTERESTED

At Newcastle University we have explored what goes on in the brain in depression but have yet to enjoy a decisive eureka moment. In an early study, we found the protein that carries serotonin in the space between nerve cells was reduced, only for a later study to contradict

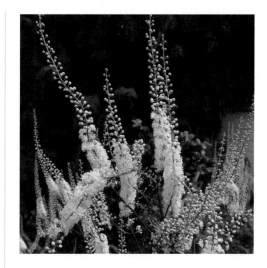

Traditional mood boosters *Crocus sativus* (saffron) **opposite** and *Actaea cimicifuga* (black cohosh) **above**.

this. We found target signals (receptors) for serotonin (such as 5HT1A and 5HT2) to be higher than normal. Then, seeking new ways, we explored a host of other brain signals (neuropeptides such as CRH, TRH, VIP, CCK), all to no avail.

Today's research for depression (and bipolar) treatment has also looked at boosting the brain's stimulatory (glutamate) signal but the buzz word is inflammation, with hopes that anti-inflammatories may be the new antidepressants. The famous St. John's wort (*Hypericum perforatum*) is as much renowned for its wound-healing and anti-inflammatory properties as for its antidepressant actions. Anti-inflammatory ingredients are common to many plants but St John's wort stands out because it was one of the first medicinal plants to be exposed to scientific review and benefit from meta-analysis covering all its controlled clinical trials. The results were published in the *British Medical Journal* (Linde et al. 1996), and this important paper did much to persuade the medical profession to take plant medicine more seriously.

There is some evidence that eating a diet rich in fruit and vegetables, which contain valuable polyphenols such as anti-inflammatory flavonoids, reduces depression. So take note of yet another reason to eat five (or perhaps more) servings a day and be aware that the plant world has the potential to provide us with remedies, and preventative strategies, for what seems to be a major epidemic in today's society. *The American Journal of Clinical Nutrition* (2016) reported that after following 82,643 women aged 53 to 80 over ten years, dietary flavonoid intake significantly lowered the risk of incidence of depression in midlife and older women across this age range (though such studies that identify trends are not necessarily indicative of cause and effect).

Below: *Hypericum perforatum* (St. John's wort) is renowned as an antidepressant and anti-inflammatory.
Opposite: Evidence is accruing for the potential of *Echium amoenum* (red feathers) to reduce depressive symptoms.

BANANAS AND DARK CHOCOLATE

It has been suggested that eating 3½ ounces (100 g) of dark chocolate or one banana has similar antidepressant effects to taking one paroxetine (SSRI) tablet. Dark chocolate is rich in polyphenols (such as the flavonoids procyanidins and epicatechins), and lab studies show these lower depressive symptoms, as does an extract of cocoa in a controlled clinical trial. Bananas are also rich in polyphenols but that's not all—they also contain tryptophan that is converted to serotonin, and in lab studies the fruit has antidepressant effects.

POTENTIAL BLUES BUSTERS

For our key blues busters we've selected eight scientifically researched, evidence-based plants and listed them in order of the strength of their scientific support, but there are many more potential blues busters accruing evidence including lavender, catnip, flowering

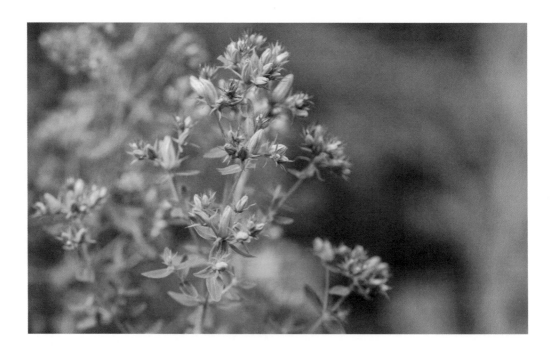

dodder, roseroot, red feathers, and rosemary. A little further out in the sidelines are *Camellia sinensis* (and its chemical catechins) and *yueju*, a Chinese herbal medicine combining five plants that is reported to deliver fast-onset clinical effectiveness for treating depression.

A tincture of lavender in combination with a conventional drug was found to be more effective than the drug alone in improving mood. An initial study has demonstrated that inhalation and massage with lavender and rose essential oil decreases depression in postpartum women and lowers premenstrual emotional symptoms. Lavender tea has been shown to lower perceived fatigue and depression in postnatal sleep-disturbed women, and when given to people taking an SSRI, it results in reduced scores of depression.

Separate studies of aromatic catnip (*Nepeta menthoides*) and the flowering dodder (*Cuscuta planiflora*) showed them as effective as conventional antidepressants in controlling mood and treating depression in people with major depression, and catnip delayed depression recurrence as well.

Roseroot (*Rhodiola rosea*) helps treat mild to moderate depression, and although not as effective as a conventional antidepressant, it has fewer side effects.

Named after its long red-flowered stems, red feathers (*Echium amoenum*) significantly reduced depressive symptoms among those with mild to moderate depression when compared with a placebo, and in a separate study reduced obsessive compulsive disorder symptoms and anxiety, too.

Rosemary (*Rosmarinus officinalis*) and lemon balm (*Melissa officinalis*) have mood-lifting effects in the lab, acting on calming (GABA) signals, and also on pleasure (dopamine) and happy (serotonin) signals.

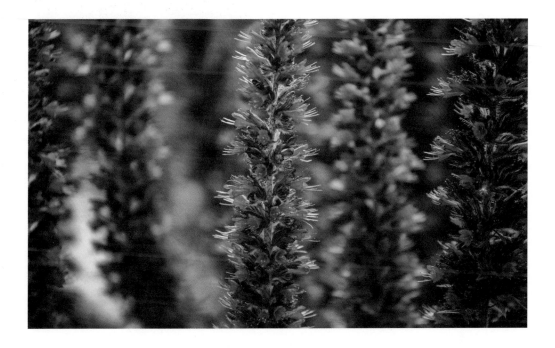

Ayahuasca (*Banisteriopsis caapi*) is an Amazonian plant that is the main constituent of a tea used in traditional rituals where it usually mixed with another plant such as chacruna (*Psychotria viridis*). The tea mix (also called ayahuasca) acts on mood-boosting signals: chacruna contains the hallucinogenic DMT (dimethyltryptamine) that activates serotonin; and ayahuasca's harmine alkaloids protect the DMT (by blocking the enzyme monoamine oxidase), which in turn increases serotonin, dopamine, and norepinephrine. Lab tests and clinical trials on the tea have so far confirmed its use as a rapid-onset antidepressant that can also reduce anxiety, alter and improve outlook, and is well tolerated.

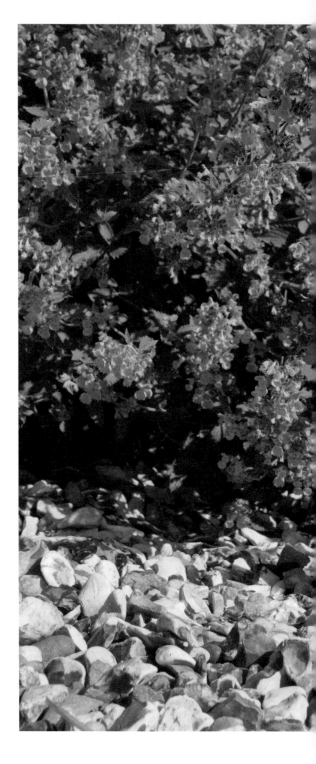

Nepeta faassenii (catnip) brings pleasure to cats, and evidence is accruing for its value as a blues buster for humans.

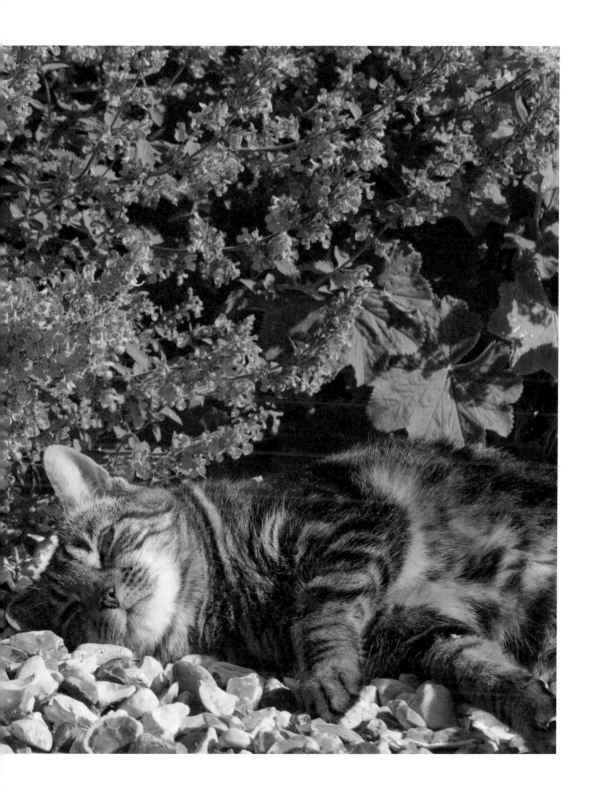

Hypericum perforatum

ST. JOHN'S WORT

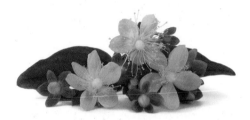

The most famous plant for mild to moderate depression and the prescribed drug of choice for medical practice in parts of Europe. It acts on a number of the brain's signals involved in depression and is also a powerful anti-inflammatory.

ABOUT THE PLANT: Native to Europe, St. John's wort is widespread and regarded as a weed. Thriving in poor chalky soil, this 31-inch (80 cm) tall perennial can behave as an annual, refusing to stay in the same area and instead self-seeding elsewhere. It has small dark green oval leaves distinguished by what look like tiny perforations that are in fact translucent oil glands. Bright yellow petals, reddish on the underside, are edged with black dots that contain its key ingredient, hypericin. It can be confused with several closely related *Hypericum* species and hybrids. The Brazilian *H. caprifoliatum* has also been investigated as an antidepressant.

HISTORY AND FOLKLORE: Known as "the blessed" in Wales, UK, and used for nervous problems in Europe, it's also been regarded as a wound healer for thousands of years. The common name comes from its tendency to flower at the solstice on St. John's Eve (June 24).

Hypericum comes from "hyper" (above) and "eikon," an image that may be unwanted (such as a ghost). In the Middle Ages the plant was thought to magically drive away demons and it's still known as "chase devil" today, recalling that one of the explanations for feeling depressed in the past was spirit possession. English herbalist John Gerard said of it, "In the world there is not a better treatment for deep wounds." It is also traditionally used in herbal medicine for nervous exhaustion, neuralgia, and menopause, and as an antiviral.

WHAT SCIENTISTS SAY: More than 700 studies since the 1980s.

In humans: Thirty clinical studies (many in Germany and Austria) show its efficacy, and in controlled trials for mild to moderate depression it is as effective as SSRIs such as Prozac, but with fewer side effects. In one Austrian study against placebo, depression improved in two-thirds of people taking St. John's wort. In other controlled studies it treats depression in menopausal women and anxiety associated with depression. Pilot studies indicate it is beneficial in physical disorders associated with stress, when used with light therapy in seasonal affective disorder (SAD), in ADHD, and in increasing deep sleep against a placebo. Its use in severe depression requires more research.

In the lab: St. John's wort affects more brain neurotransmitters and hormones (such as serotonin, dopamine, monoamine oxidase, GABA, glutamate as well as acetylcholine, opioid, noradrenaline, and melatonin) that affect mood, among other things, than do SSRIs. It is also anti-inflammatory, pain relieving and neuroprotective (such as antiamyloid).

A study in Switzerland showed that St. John's wort extract taken for a year effectively halved two measures of depression in 440 people with mild to moderate depression.

KEY INGREDIENTS: Hypericin, hyperforin and adhyperforin (naphthodianthrones) may be responsible for antidepressant effects, though the whole extract is considered essential. Hypericin on its own boosts mood. It contains flavonoids (such as quercetin) and also nicotine. Its essential oil contains the calming and cognition-boosting pinenes (also in lavender and pine).

HOW TO TAKE IT: Take a tincture of 150 g fresh plant per 500 ml of 40% alcohol 2.5 ml 3 times daily. Buy capsules or tablets. Makes a not unpleasant, woody but bitter tea of leaves and flowers. Also infuse flowers in olive oil and use essential oil in aromatherapy.

SAFETY: Adverse effects rare at normal doses. Nausea and phototoxicity occasionally reported. Caution with around 50 percent of conventional drugs such as immunosuppressants, cardiovasculars, chemotherapeuticals and contraceptives—hyperforin turns on genes for common drug metabolizing enzymes (for example CYT3A4) in the intestine, and the liver therefore renders many drugs less effective. Caution with antianxiety, antidepressant (especially SSRIs), and antipsychotic drugs and at high quantity with valerian. Not enough information to predict safety in pregnancy. St. John's wort is on the UK Traditional Herbal Registration for low mood and anxiety.

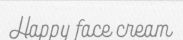

Happy face cream

Wake up and go to sleep with happiness in a jar! This lovely cream lifts the mood as the essential oil constituents permeate the skin. Use a commercial base face lotion that is either organic or contains natural ingredients. Mix in pure St. John's wort essential oil to a proportion not exceeding 1% of the entire mixture.

After thorough mixing, store the cream in dark brown or black jars. Label clearly with an image of the bright yellow flower. When using, inhale deeply as you massage it over your face.

Turmeric-spiced fish curry

Serves 6

1 tablespoon fennel seeds, toasted

1 tablespoon yellow mustard seeds, toasted

1 teaspoon ground coriander

1 teaspoon ground cumin

1 long red chile pepper, sliced

1 tablesppon coarsely chopped fresh ginger

2 tablespoons coarsely chopped fresh turmeric

2 tablespoons vegetable oil

14-ounce (400 ml) can coconut milk

2¼ pounds (1 kg) firm white fish fillets, cut into large chunks

1 tablespoon fresh lime juice

Handful of cilantro leaves, chopped

Don't be put off by the long list of ingredients— there are only five steps to this fresh, blues-busting fish curry.

❶ Grind the fennel and mustard seeds with a pestle and mortar and add the coriander and cumin.

❷ Place the chile, ginger and turmeric in a small food processor and blend until you have a fine paste. Combine with the dry spices.

❸ Heat the oil in a large, shallow saucepan and stir-fry the spice paste over a high heat for 2 to 3 minutes, until it gives off good aromas.

❹ Add the coconut milk and bring to a boil. Simmer for 8 to 10 minutes, until reduced to a thick, creamy sauce.

❺ Add the fish to the pan and cook for 7 minutes or until cooked through. Add the lime juice and freshly ground pepper to taste.

❻ Serve with steamed rice and a garnish of cilantro leaves and grated turmeric.

Curcuma longa syn. *C. domestica*

TURMERIC

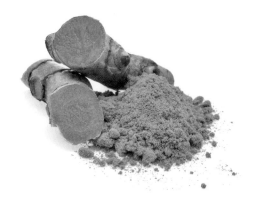

This beautiful tropical plant, holy and auspicious in India, has been used for thousands of years from kitchen to clinic. Best known as a major ingredient of curry, it improves mood and has multiple other health benefits, many scientifically verified.

ABOUT THE PLANT: A perennial from South Asia that likes humid conditions and well-drained soil, it has long, blade-like, bunched, sweet-smelling leaves and star-like yellow and pink flower heads. A member of the ginger family growing to 39 inches (1 m), its rhizome (harvested in winter) looks similar to ginger but beneath the skin its flesh is bright yellow/orange with a peppery aroma and mild, sweet flavor. In temperate zones it grows well in pots indoors.

HISTORY AND FOLKLORE: Listed in Assyrian herbals from 600 BC and used by Dioscorides in the first century AD, its name comes from *tarmaret* (Latin *terra merita*, merit of the earth). Hindu monks' robes are dyed in turmeric to reflect the "sun solar

plexus chakra." Traditionally used in Asia (it's a major ingredient in the medicine Xioyao-san) and in Europe for stress, depression, as an anti-inflammatory and anticoagulant. Today, research into turmeric is expanding as the interest in food as medicine is reawakened in the West.

WHAT SCIENTISTS SAY

In humans: The plant extract or its ingredient curcumin improve mood in major depression in several controlled trials. It is a powerful anti-inflammatory (tested stronger than hydrocortisone), reduces inflammation (C-reactive protein) in some controlled studies, and alleviates pain. It also improves memory in pilot controlled trials, quality of life in cancer patients due to suppressing tumour-related inflammation, and is clinically antioxidant. Over 100 clinical trials show its efficacy in chronic disease from cancers, diabetes, and obesity to cardiovascular, pulmonary, autoimmune, and neurological conditions. It's bioavailability (being insoluble in water) may have limited some clinical trial outcomes.

The first clinical study to show curcumin effective for depression was in Gujarat, India. There, curcumin was given for six weeks to 60 people with major depression. It was found to be as effective, in two assessment measures, as the conventional (SSRI) antidepressant fluoxetine.

In the lab: Numerous preclinical studies show a potential role for curcumin in bipolar disorder and post-traumatic stress disorder. It alters neuronal growth in models of stress and is antidepressant and neuroprotective in several models. Like rosemary, curcumin boosts the memory signal (acetylcholine) and brain dopamine and interacts with stimulatory (glutamate) and mood-boosting serotonin. Essential oil constituent bisabolene is anticonvulsant, and turmeric improves memory in lab models.

KEY INGREDIENTS: The bioactive yellow curcumin (60 percent of its polyphenol content) has been extensively investigated and affects various molecules and systems. The essential oil contains bisabolene, limonene, and curcumene (also in lemon verbena). Its unusual aroma is due to turmerone, arturmerone, and zingiberene.

HOW TO TAKE IT: Root freshly grated or dried can be taken as a tea up to 1 g daily or tincture (150 g fresh per 500 ml) 1 teaspoon 3 times daily. Adds distinctive flavor freshly grated in salads. Used in cooking, in almost any dish, fat is added to help absorption. Taken dried as powder (4 g) in food or mixed with water or milk (2 times daily; adding 1 teaspoon lecithin may help absorption). Tablets or capsules (some commercial preparations claim better bioavailability) or essential oil.

SAFETY: No adverse effects at recommended dose. Higher doses may cause gastrointestinal effects. Contraindicated in biliary obstruction. May interact with anticoagulants, antidepressants, antibiotics, chemotherapeutic agents, antihistamines, and other anti-inflammatory drugs where doses greater than 15 g per day should not be used. Avoid sun with topical application as is found phototoxic in the lab. Can be adulterated with lead oxide or an illegal yellow dye. Caution when handling as removing yellow stains is challenging.

Crocus sativus

SAFFRON

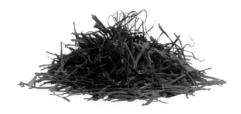

Saffron really is a mellow yellow. This delicate flower (and the world's most expensive spice) significantly reduces symptoms of depression in clinical trials.

ABOUT THE PLANT: Spanish saffron or parrot's corn is a bulbous perennial native to India and the eastern Mediterranean, with narrow leaves and pretty purple blooms, each with three deep red stigmas. Harvested in early autumn and dried, it takes a quarter of a million hand-picked stigmas and 1 acre (0.4 hectare) of land to make a pound of spice. It used to be cultivated near the town of Saffron Walden in the UK, named accordingly.

HISTORY AND FOLKLORE: On the island of Santorini in Greece is a fresco dated 1600 BC showing young women gathering saffron for what may be a medical use. In folklore you burn or carry it for healing, where it's said to strengthen psychic awareness. There are also remarkable 50,000-year-old drawings in northwest Iran that use saffron-based pigments. Its name comes from the Arabic for yellow (*zafran*), and it was highly valued as a culinary spice, dye, and medicine by the Greeks and Romans. In Western herbal medicine it is used to counter depression, calm nerves, induce sleep in insomniacs, and for shock and neuralgia. "Saffron has power to quicken the spirits . . . provoking laughter and merriment," wrote the herbalist Christopher Catton in 1862.

WHAT SCIENTISTS SAY

In humans: Pooling all results in a meta-analysis of several randomized, high-quality controlled trials, there are highly significant effects of saffron supplementation on mild and moderate depressive symptoms, showing it is as effective as current antidepressant medications (both tricyclic and SSRIs) and without the side effects of conventional medications. Petals work as well as the stigmas. Its key ingredient crocin on its own is also effective, but not as well tolerated. Saffron is also shown in controlled trials to counter cognitive decline in Alzheimer's as effectively as the Alzheimer's drug memantine. Saffron also clinically treats premenstrual tension and sexual dysfunction in females taking antidepressants.

Tehran University conducted a controlled trial involving saffron petals and 40 people with major depression. They were given either a capsule of the dried petal (15 mg) or the standard SSRI antidepressant fluoxetine (10 mg), morning and evening. After eight weeks, saffron was found to be as effective as fluoxetine in the treatment of mild to moderate depression.

In the lab: Saffron counters obsessive compulsive disorder (OCD) and works on the mood-boosting (serotonin) and reward (dopamine) signals, and also affects memory (acetylcholine), excitatory (glutamate), and neuroendocrine pathways as well as being anti-inflammatory.

KEY INGREDIENTS: Saffron's major chemicals are the bitter crocin (a deep red carotenoid) and safranal (in the essential oil), which give its aroma. Crocin increases serotonin and dopamine—it blocks the enzyme monoamine oxidase and is a potent neuronal antioxidant, too.

HOW TO TAKE IT: Medical herbalists recommend 1 g of raw plant a day—that's 150 flowers, which makes it too expensive for watery teas or traditional tinctures, but good for adding a unique flavor to salads, paellas, and stews. Saffron capsules, tablets, and tinctures are also available, as are tablets of its key active ingredient crocin.

SAFETY: No significant side effects reported, but beware nausea at higher doses. Caution with other antidepressant medication can be extrapolated, however there is no evidence for this. Can be adulterated with turmeric, capsicum, marigold, or safflower. Do not take large doses in pregnancy.

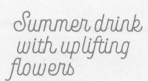

Summer drink with uplifting flowers

Add sprigs of beautiful blue borage, St John's wort, clary sage, and especially saffron flowers to gin and tonic, wine cup, Pimms, or elderflower cordial.

Get muddy, get happy!

A study at the University of Colorado showed the harmless bacteria *Mycobacterium vaccae*, found in soil, may act as a natural antidepressant (anti-inflammatory) in the lab. The bacteria create an immune response that affects the release and metabolism of serotonin in parts of the brain controlling cognitive function and mood. So don't scrub those organic carrots and potatoes so hard, and encourage children to get muddy and increase their microbiome! While you're outside, take a walk, bike, or run to pump up your brain's endorphins, those feel-good neurotransmitters that keep athletes going.

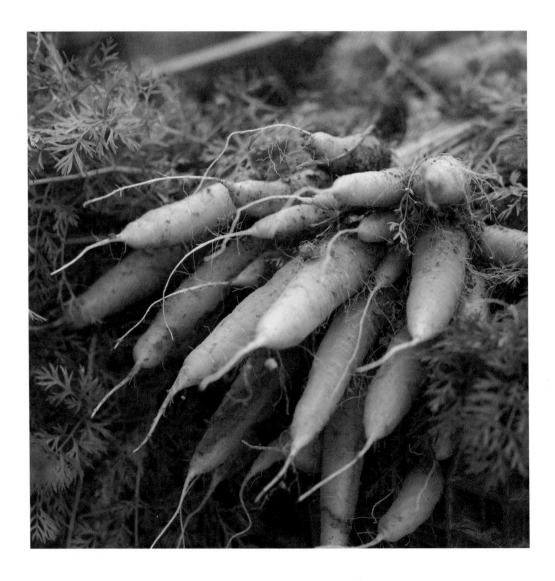

Actaea racemosa syn. *Cimicifuga racemosa*

BLACK COHOSH

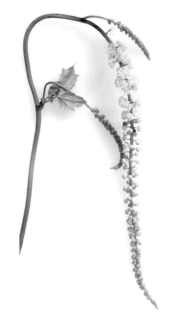

The reputation of this plant for mental health related to hormonal changes in women has spread throughout the world as a result of its use by Native Americans.

ABOUT THE PLANT: A perennial native to the USA and southwest Canada and now wild in Europe. Grows up to 8 feet 3 inches (2.5 m), preferring shade. Deep cut three-point leaves and dramatic long, white, sweetly scented flowers, consisting only of stamens and stigmas (having no petals or sepals). It produces a dry black fruit with many seeds. Also called squaw root, the rhizome is dark brown/black, knobbly, and hairy. Roots are harvested in autumn after aerial parts have died down.

HISTORY AND FOLKLORE: Known as fairy candle and black or rattle snakeroot (it was used to treat snakebite), cohosh is considered a "miracle herb" for women by Native Americans who have used it for gynecological complaints and as a normalizer of the female reproductive system for the past 100 years. It is said to balance hormones and mood swings and lessen anxiety associated with hormonal changes in women (PMT, postnatal and menopause). Used in herbal medicine as an analgesic (anti-inflammatory) and for painful or delayed menstruation, ovarian cramps, sciatica, neuralgia, and as a sedative. Other cohosh species are used in Chinese herbal medicine for headaches.

WHAT SCIENTISTS SAY

In humans: Studies (many in Germany) show black cohosh is effective in treating depression. In controlled studies it significantly enhances the effects of conventional antidepressants (SSRIs), is as effective as the hormone oestrogen in reducing depression (and also improves fertility). Other studies show black cohosh reduces anxiety, irritability, and hot flushes in menopausal women and improves sleep quality in postmenopausal women but more research is warranted to overcome variations in study design and plant extract.

In 2005, Pavia University in Italy compared the steroid estradiol to black cohosh in 64 women and found that both produced an identical and significant reduction in anxiety and depression after three months.

In the lab: Works on pleasure and reward signals (serotonin, dopamine and noradrenaline). The alkaloid methyl-serotonin may be responsible for antidepressive effects. The extract is hormone modulating, suppressing luteinizing hormone (LH), thereby increasing progesterone production. Glycosides reduce osteoporosis.

KEY INGREDIENTS: Anemonin. Triterpene saponins (also known as bitter glycosides) such as aceteol and cimigenol. Also contains aromatic acids (such as ferulic acid), resins, and salicylic acid.

HOW TO TAKE IT: Harvested in autumn, use the dried rather than fresh root, as the ingredient ranunculin changes to the key bioctive anemonin. Decoction (20 g chopped dried root per 750 ml water simmered to 500 ml) 120 ml 2 times daily, tastes bitter but seems to be a preferred way to take it (in menopause). Tincture, capsules, and tablets also used.

SAFETY: Well tolerated. Do not take in pregnancy or breastfeeding. Caution in some hormone-sensitive disorders. Although a member of the buttercup family, it has no such toxicity. Caution in liver disease, though controlled trials do not support reports of liver damage. At higher doses nausea and dizziness can rarely occur. Not to be confused with blue cohosh (*Caulophyllum thalictroides*), also called squaw vine, a blue-berried member of the barberry family, used as an abortive and contraceptive. Black cohosh is on the UK Traditional Herbal Registration for relief of symptoms of menopause.

Scutellaria lateriflora

SKULLCAP

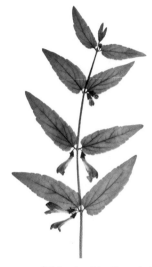

The name of this plant in the mint family alludes to its use. It packs some punch in its traditional role of treating nervous disorders and there is growing clinical evidence backing its ability to lift the mood.

ABOUT THE PLANT: Small, slow-growing to 39 inches (1 m), this many-branched perennial has few nondescript paired leaves and tiny skull-like seed heads (Latin *scutella* means dish). Native to eastern USA, it is at home in marshes and wetlands and is found all over North America. The blue, helmet-shaped flowers have gained it the names blue pimpernel, helmet flower, and hoodwort. The roots of the Asian species (*Scutellaria baicalensis*) and the South American species (*Scutellaria indica* f. *racemosa*) are used for cognitive disorders. The species used in Western herbal medicine is *S. lateriflora* where aerial parts are harvested during flowering. It tastes bitter and astringent.

HISTORY AND FOLKLORE: People bathed in skullcap leaves, or used them to cast spells to remove disharmony. Its other name of mad-dog herb relates to it being used to treat rabies in the nineteenth century (though evidence for this is lacking). Discovered in the nineteenth century as a nervous system tonic, it's used to treat depression, panic attacks, and nervous heart conditions. One of the most popular botanicals in North America (the Cherokee use it for menstrual nervous problems), in herbal medicine it's used for depression, as a relaxant, mild sedative, sleep promoter, and to help in withdrawal of benzodiazepines. A mood modifier not only for humans, it's used by vets to help calm dogs suffering from excitability, apprehension, and phobias such as fear of thunderstorms and gunfire (and there's no drowsiness or reduction in performance—perfect for training and obedience).

WHAT SCIENTISTS SAY

In humans: In one "gold standard" controlled study, skullcap showed significant effects on mood in healthy volunteers. After two weeks, mood was significantly enhanced, without reduction in energy or cognition. Its ingredient baicalein has been tested in volunteers (with a view to treating people with Parkinson's disease) and found to be safe and well tolerated.

American skullcap (Scutellaria lateriflora) significantly boosted mood in 43 volunteers in a "gold standard" trial—a randomized, double-blind placebo-controlled crossover study.

In the lab: Whole extracts and its key ingredient baicalein are antidepressive and anti-inflammatory in a number of models and affect the hypothalamic-pituitary-adrenal axis. Acts on the serotonin signal (stops LSD binding) and prevents an Alzheimer's marker. Also acts on calming (GABA benzodiazepine) signals and is antianxiety and anticonvulsant.

KEY INGREDIENTS: Flavonoids baicalin, baicalein and scutellarin are key to antidepressive effects and keeping inflammation at bay in a wide range of lab tests and are also key antioxidants, scavenging free radicals. Ingredient wogonin is neuroregenerative and baicalein is neuroprotective. Also contains melatonin and serotonin.

HOW TO TAKE IT: Tea of fresh (4 to 6 g) or dried (2 to 3 g) aerial parts per 240 ml water, take 50 ml 3 times daily. Tincture, capsules, or tablets (and of its key ingredient baicalein) are also used.

SAFETY: Generally regarded as safe. Side effects are drowsiness, giddiness, confusion. Overdose may cause convulsions. Always buy from a reputable source—there are disturbing reports in the 1980s that many commercial products did not contain any skullcap and were adulterated with other plants such as germander (*Teucrium chamaedrys*) and other *Teucrium* species which can cause hepatotoxicity. Do not take in pregnancy and lactation. Sedative effects on nervous system mean it may interact with other antidepressants, sedatives, or anesthetics.

Sunbathe and day-dream

The sun makes us feel good and sunbathing near a brightly colored blues buster like St. John's wort or crocus can only enhance the sensation. Phototherapy (treatment with artificial light) is clinically effective for those who experience SAD (seasonal affective disorder). The increased levels of vitamin D also lift mood and help sleep. If you can get your sunlight off-grid and in nature, this is even better as it lowers your heart rate and relaxes the body.

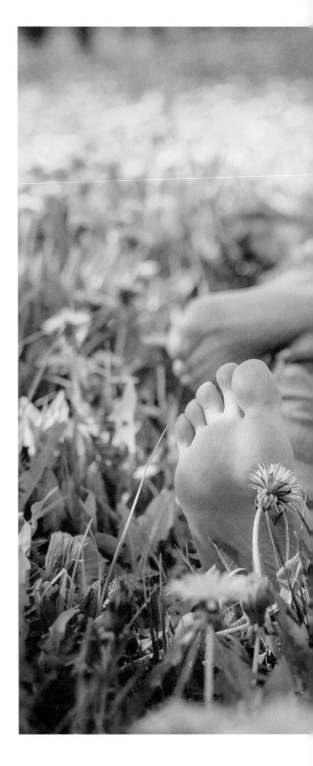

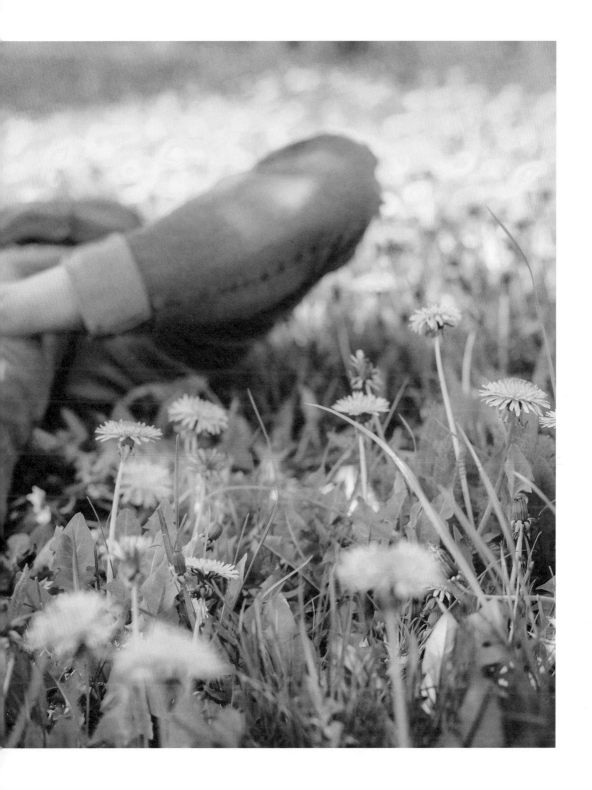

Salvia sclarea

CLARY SAGE

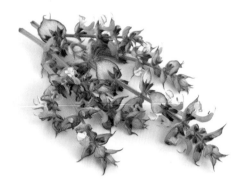

Favored by aromatherapists, clary sage has scientifically confirmed antidepressant and pain-relieving actions and is renowned in helping female hormonal conditions, both physical and mental.

ABOUT THE PLANT: A beautiful biennial native to Europe and the Middle East, it is cultivated in Russia and France for its mood-lifting essential oil. Preferring a dry sunny site, it grows to 39 inches (1 m), with wrinkly, hairy leaves and whorls of pale blue-purple flowers.

HISTORY AND FOLKLORE: In folklore it is an aphrodisiac and induces euphoria. The Romans brought clary to the UK for rituals to deities such as Luna and Diana. People still write their wishes on leaves, put them under the pillow, and hope they will come true. Also called clear eye and see bright—traditionally the seed's mucilaginous coating is used to remove objects from eyes and to treat eye problems (sclarea comes from Latin *clarus*, meaning clear). Used in herbal medicine as an antidepressant, calming tonic and also to relieve menstrual pain, premenstrual problems, menopausal complaints, and as an estrogenic. Its essential oil is considered by aromatherapists to lift mood and be the most relaxing of all essential oils, and is widely used for anxiety, as a sedative, antispasmodic, anticonvulsant, and hypotensive. Cultivated for its ingredient sclareol (from which ambrox, found in ambergris, can be synthesized), which is used in perfume and flavoring, including vermouth.

WHAT SCIENTISTS SAY

In humans: Preliminary studies show antidepressive effects in 22 menopausal women after inhalation of the aromatic oil, where it decreased cortisol and raised serotonin in the blood. The change was more significant in those already depressed, who rated improvements in mood, too. In a separate study inhalation lowered blood pressure (diastolic and systolic). The essential oil, applied topically, in combination with lavender, rose (*Rosa centifolia*), and/or marjoram (*Origanum majorana*), decreased pain in menstrual cramps in students (in a controlled study) and decreased pain in labor.

In the lab: Essential oil is antidepressant and antianxiety, acting at the content (serotonin) and pleasure (dopamine) brain signals. The antidepressive potency was found to be greater than chamomile, rosemary, and lavender and comparable to the chemical fluoxetine. Also protective in stress-induced cardiovascular models, antioxidant, and neuroprotective.

KEY INGREDIENTS: Essential oil contains linalool and linalyl acetate, two ingredients in lavender that reduce anxiety and depression in lab models (via glutamate, serotonin, and dopamine brain signals), and which together with ingredients cineole and caryophyllene are pain relieving. Oil also contains terpineol and the diterpenes sclareol and farnesene—the latter is also present in the calming chamomile (*Matricaria recutita*).

HOW TO TAKE IT: Essential oil commonly used in aromatherapy. Tea, called "misk sage" is popular in Turkey.

SAFETY: Do not take in pregnancy.

Bupleurum chinense

CHAI HU

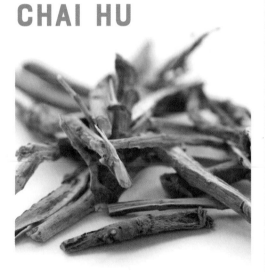

This traditional Chinese medicine for "harmony" is a mild sedative often used in a combination that clinically improves mood in depressed, insomniac women.

ABOUT THE PLANT: This perennial 39 inches (1 m) tall plant is in the carrot family and needs copious sun and well-drained soil. It resembles fennel or dill in its yellow flower clusters in autumn, and has long sickle-shaped leaves ("hare's ears"). It is the long, brown, branched, wrinkly root (up to 8 inches/20 cm) of *Bupleurum chinense* that is considered the original chai hu (pharmaceutical name in Chinese herbal medicine is *Radix bupleuri*) but other species are used, including *B. falcatumv* in Japan. One related species is toxic (*B. longiradiatum*).

HISTORY AND FOLKLORE: Called thorowax root, *chai hu* (China), *saiko* (Japan), *segl-hareøre* (Danish) and hare's ear root (UK), this plant is commonly used in Chinese herbal medicine in combinations. Used since the first century BC for fever, pain, dizziness, debility, and emotional instability. Also a primary part of Japanese (Kampo) medicine today and a common medicine for insomnia in Taiwan.

WHAT SCIENTISTS SAY

In humans: Initial pilot studies, in combination with cinnamon and ginger, showed chai hu clinically improved mood in 90 depressed insomniac females, and lowered measures of inflammation. Widely studied in several universities in Japan (such as the Faculty of Medicine, Miyazaki University) in combination with six other medicinal plants that make up the Japanese medicine *yokukansan*, it clinically improves behavioral symptoms such as irritability, anxiety, apathy, delusions, hallucinations, and psychosis (in autism-related disorders), in schizophrenia (controlled study), Parkinson's, Alzheimer's, vascular and Lewy body dementia.

In the lab: Extracts and saikosaponins are antidepressant, sedative and antiepileptic in several lab models. Saikosaponins stop the stimulatory actions of caffeine and methamphetamine. Affects reward (dopamine and noradrenaline) signals.

KEY INGREDIENTS: Saikosides/saikosaponins (triterpene saponins) show sedative effects in the lab. Also contains bioactive bupleurumol, flavonoids, and coumarins. Essential oil from the root contains 30 percent hexanal (also in olives and pears), the aroma of freshly cut grass.

HOW TO TAKE IT: In China, the ground dried root of chai hu is used at the daily dose of 3 to 9 g by decoction. The root is cooked in boiling water (decoction 15 g in 750 ml) to make tea or soup 250 ml 3 times daily.

SAFETY: May increase effects of central nervous system (CNS) depressants (sedatives and tranquilizers). Large doses produce drowsiness and may increase bowel movements. Overdose causes nausea and vomiting and liver damage. Caution: one related species is toxic (*Bupleurum longiradiatum*).

Rosa gallica var. *officinalis, Rosa canina*

APOTHECARY'S ROSE, DOG ROSE

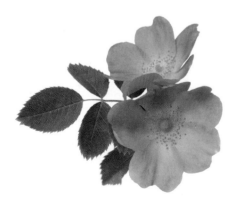

A much-loved garden plant, the rose is being rediscovered for health and well-being as a result of scientific research on the aromatic oil. The apothecary's rose is a hybrid of *Rosa centifolia* (Provence rose) and *R. canina* (dog rose). Hips, used traditionally, continue to provide benefits that are science based.

ABOUT THE PLANT: Apothecary's rose is a perennial shrub growing to 5 feet (1.5m), with sharp thorns, serrated leaves, and delicately scented, deep pink flowers. Native to the Middle East, it's been cultivated around the world for centuries. Hybridization of the apothecary's rose gave rise to the strongly scented damask rose (*Rosa × damascena*) and Provence rose (*Rosa centifolia*) from which essential oils are commonly extracted. The dog rose (*R. canina*) with sweet-scented white or pink flowers and more delicate stems and sharp thorns is found in the wild and self-seeds. Neither need much attention except to control their tendency to spread.

HISTORY AND FOLKLORE: Renowned for lifting the spirits, this queen of flowers is used in folklore to make or mend alliances, and as an aphrodisiac. Used by the Romans in festivities where petals were eaten, roses were valued in monastic gardens both spiritually, as symbols of Christ's blood, and for their healing powers. Traditionally used as an antidepressant—the first-century Arab physician Avicenna prepared rose water, while sixteenth-century British herbalist John Gerard said, "The distilled water is good for the strengthening of the heart, and refreshing of the spirits, and likewise for all things that require a gentle cooling." Hips are used as a sedative in herbal medicine and the essential oil ("attar of rose") is used in aromatherapy as an antidepressant, a sedative, and for pain relief in arthritis.

WHAT SCIENTISTS SAY

In humans: Initial studies show rose scent increases measures of parasympathetic (rest) activity and induces feelings of contentment. Essential oil relieves anxiety during labor and depression and (with lavender) anxiety in postpartum women. It relieves pain in children, menstruation, lower back and migraine in controlled trials. It improves sleep quality in coronary care patients and sexual function (in males and females) in major depression. Rose water reduced anxiety in renal patients and hips improved wellness ratings and lower blood pressure and back pain in other pilot studies.

In the lab: The petals, essential oil, and hips (wild, *R. canina*) are antidepressant, antianxiety, anticonvulsant, hypnotic, analgesic, and neuroprotective in lab tests.

KEY INGREDIENTS: The expensive pure essential oil is a mix of plant terpenes including the calming and uplifting citronellol, geraniol, linalool (also in lavender), and nerol (also in bitter orange). As with lemon balm oil, beware of imitations spiked with other cheaper oils or chemicals. Hips contain flavonoids and polyphenols.

HOW TO TAKE IT: The essential oil is commonly used in aromatherapy. Rose buds make one of the best botanical teas, fresh rose petals can be added to salads and hips make perfect jellies and syrups to eat on toast or with cheese or red meats. Rose water (extract of flowers) can be used in cocktails such as gin fizz.

SAFETY: Buds, petals, hips, and essential oil in diffusers are safe, including for children.

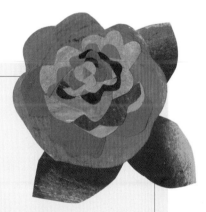

Mindfulness among the roses

Take time out to walk round a bed of roses in the park or dab a few drops of rose otto essential oil on your desk and have a break from work. Do nothing but concentrate on your sensations—any sound you might hear, the colors and shapes you see. If your mind wanders (and it will) just bring it back to your breath and to the sensations around you, again and again. It's all about concentrating on the here and now and slowing continuous circular thoughts.

Mindfulness-based cognitive therapy has been shown to relieve depression in premenstrual syndrome in women, veterans with post-traumatic stress disorder, college students with attention deficit hyperactivity disorder, and clinically depressed patients (whose sleep quality also improves).

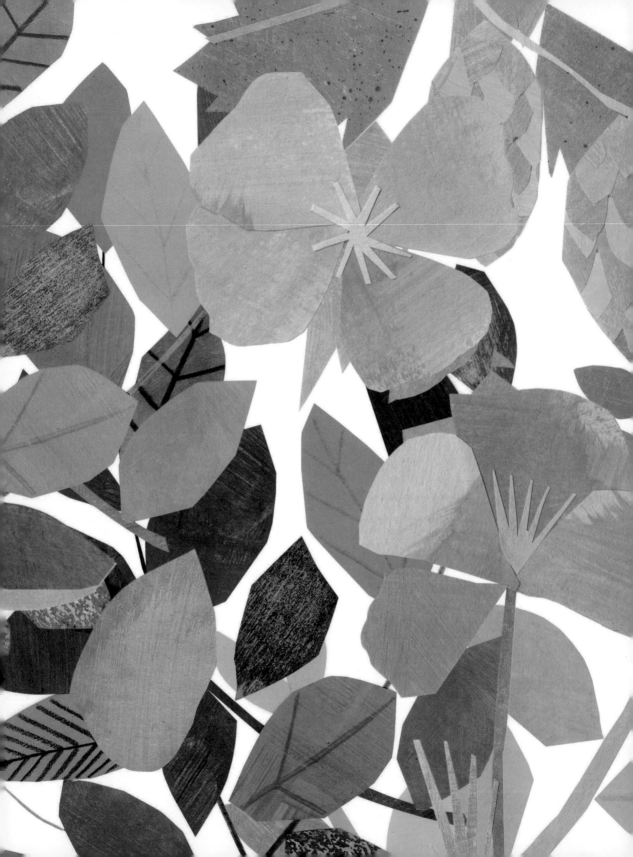

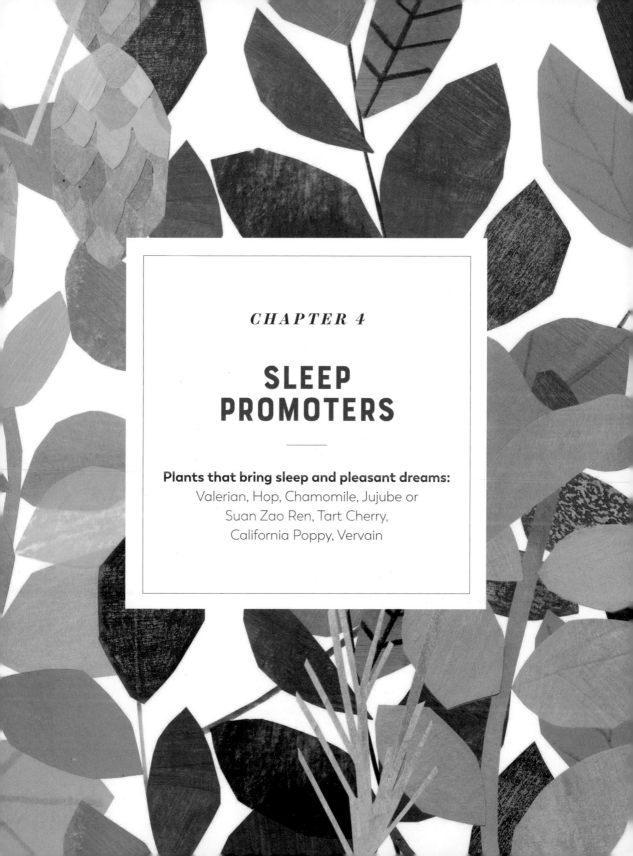

CHAPTER 4

SLEEP PROMOTERS

Plants that bring sleep and pleasant dreams:
Valerian, Hop, Chamomile, Jujube or
Suan Zao Ren, Tart Cherry,
California Poppy, Vervain

We all feel better after a good night's sleep and recognize the difference it makes to our mental and physical well-being—recent research shows that our memory is improved by a restful sleep too—but sleep problems are common and many of us reach for solutions. Insomnia is the most common sleep disorder but there are others that affect sleep to a dangerous degree, such as sleep apnea which interferes with breathing, and rapid eye movement (REM) sleep disorder in which people act out their dreams. Then there is chronic insomnia, which affects 15 percent of us, and transient sleeplessness (disrupted nighttime sleep for no more than two weeks duration), which affects up to 80 percent of us.

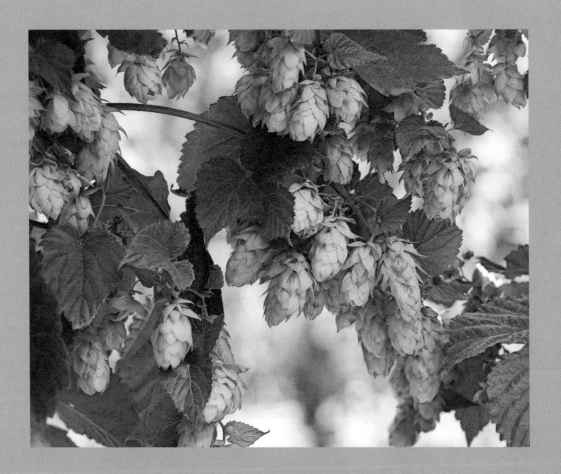

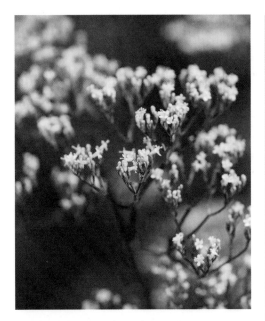

Above: *Valeriana officinalis* (valerian) alone and in combination with *Humulus lupulus* (hop) **opposite** significantly enhances sleep.

Orthodox sleep medicines are among the most commonly prescribed drugs today and usually include benzodiazepines, sedating antidepressants, antiepileptics, and over-the-counter sedating antihistamines. Chemical hypnotics (agents that make you sleep) are not always ideal, especially in the long term because they bring with them "hangover" side effects, aftereffects, and dependency. A recent meta-analysis of conventional drugs used to treat insomnia concluded that while they may improve short-term sleep outcomes, their "comparative effectiveness and long-term efficacy are not known and may cause cognitive and behavioral changes, and are associated with infrequent but serious harms" (such as falls).

WHAT GOES ON IN THE BRAIN?

Brain mechanisms enmeshed in sleep and dreaming are complex, and many signals are implicated, the best known of which is melatonin. Another, adenosine, builds up in the brain during the day to make us feel sleepy. Adenosine inhibits wakefulness processes in the body, involving other signals such as norepinephrine, acetylcholine, and serotonin, and is reduced by caffeine. Other sleep brain signals and pathways are GABA (the calming signal), opiates and cannabinoids (pain), and dopamine (drive and pleasure). Agents that boost these brain signals often induce sleep at lower doses and intensify dreaming at higher doses. The fascinating but sometimes frightening dreams induced by opium poppy described in Thomas De Quincey's *Confessions of an English Opium-Eater* in 1821 were the results of dangerously high doses.

THE SCIENCE OF DREAMING

Closely associated with sleep are the mysteries of dreams and dreaming. Some people claim they never dream at all, while others are acutely aware of their dreams and regularly refer to them. But neither the philosophers of old nor scientists of today can agree on why we dream. Whether it's rapid eye movement (REM) or non-REM sleep, there's no doubt that mental activity, remembered or not, takes place throughout most of the sleep cycle—and surveys suggest dream content is more likely to be the anxious or worried kind rather than happy and relaxed.

This last observation struck the renowned dream researcher Alan Hobson as crucial. At a meeting devoted to dreaming, held halfway up a mountainside in the Italian Alps, we presented our research findings on hallucinations and speculated on how these might relate to dreaming. We were clear that, whatever its function, not being allowed to dream (dream deprivation) actually leads to hallucinations. But Alan seized center stage when he

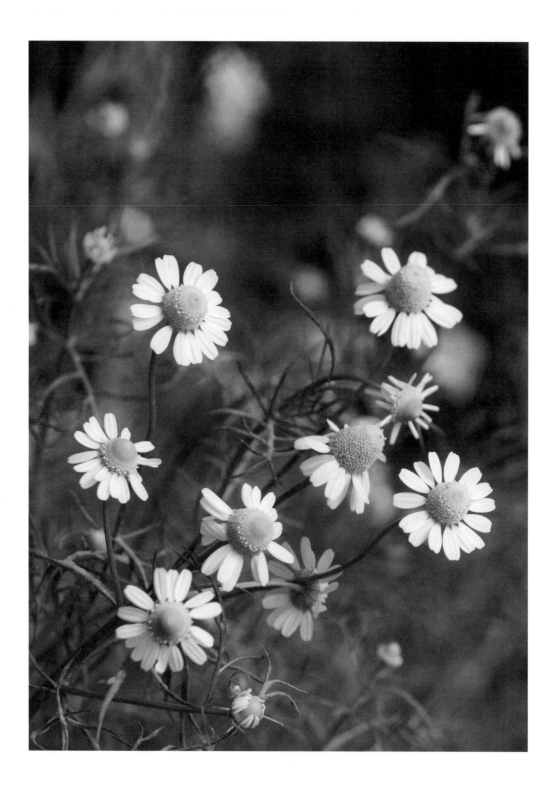

YOUR BRAIN ON PLANTS

announced his latest theory, which is that dreaming is a survival mechanism and that we need to regularly run our minds through virtual scenarios in order to more easily deal with the unsettling or dangerous dramas that confront us in real life.

BOTANICAL SLEEP BALMS

In view of the side effects from and risk of dependency on orthodox sleep medicines, whole plant sedatives, which are effective and nonaddictive, have a widespread appeal— not least since they have a higher margin of safety than conventional drugs. We highlight seven plants which science demonstrates are promoters of sleep in order of the most scientific backing to the least. Foremost is valerian, an established hypnotic plant with strong safety and efficacy credentials for treating insomnia, closely followed by hop. Many studies show valerian (alone or in combination with hop) significantly enhances sleep. Other key plants to improve depth, duration, and quality of sleep are chamomile, jujube, tart cherry, California poppy, and vervain.

Sleep-inducing brain balms included in other chapters are gotu kola, passionflower and ashwagandha, skullcap, cannabis, wild lettuce, catnip, and the classic, lavender. Nighttime teas or tinctures, aromatherapy, or botanical pillows made from these medicinal plants have all been shown to be effective.

Opposite: *Chamaemelum nobile* (chamomile) improves the depth, duration, and quality of sleep.
Above: *Cananga odorata* (ylang-ylang) has traditionally been used as a sleep promoter in the Far East but has yet to be explored by science.

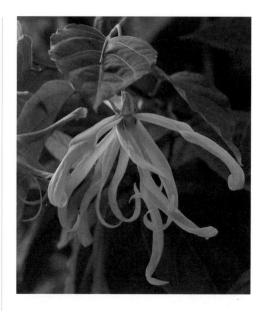

ALPHA-PINENE

Alpha-pinene is a chemical found in the essential oils of many aromatic stress-busting plants including pine, cannabis, sage, frankincense, and valerian. When you inhale the pine needle–like aroma, the small molecule alpha-pinene reaches your brain to calm by enhancing inhibitory (GABA) signals. It also enhances the first stages of non-REM sleep.

TRADITIONAL SLEEP PROMOTERS

There are many more plants traditionally used to induce sleep that haven't yet been fully explored by science. For example, Jamaican dogwood (*Piscidia piscipula*), Indian mulberry (*Morinda citrifolia*), mulungu or coral flower (*Erythrina mulungu*), a powerful traditional sedative plant from Brazil and Peru, and Mediterranean cedar (*Cedrus*). From the Far East there is chrysanthemum (*Chrysanthemum morifolium*), ylang-ylang (*Cananga odorata*), magnolia (*Magnolia officinalis*), gardenia (*Gardenia jasminoides*), and schisandra (*Schisandra chinensis*).

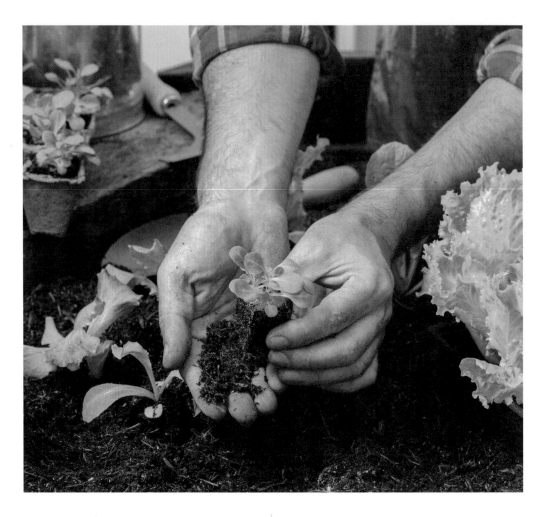

SLEEP BALM CONTENDERS

The following four plants have attracted some scientific support.

Lettuce (*Lactuca sativa*) is backed by abundant evidence for its sleep-inducing properties, which are concentrated in the white latex in its stems. A clinical trial shows the seeds have safe sleep-inducing effects, thought to be due to chemicals such as lactucin which are sedative but nonaddictive, and also in wild lettuce (*L. virosa*)

Lotus (*Nelumbo nucifera*) figures in Greek mythology. Odysseus met the lotus eaters living on an island abundant in lotus plants that induced such deep sleep that he and his men had to be carried back to their ship. Lab studies of lotus ingredients (alkaloids like liensinine) show they induce sleep in lab models by controlling the brain's calming signal.

Wuling is one of many traditional Chinese medicines for insomnia, and more than 200 clinical trials from the East back up their traditional use. While study methods have been criticized by some for lack of rigor, the indications are that the Chinese medicines have fewer side effects than Western drugs.

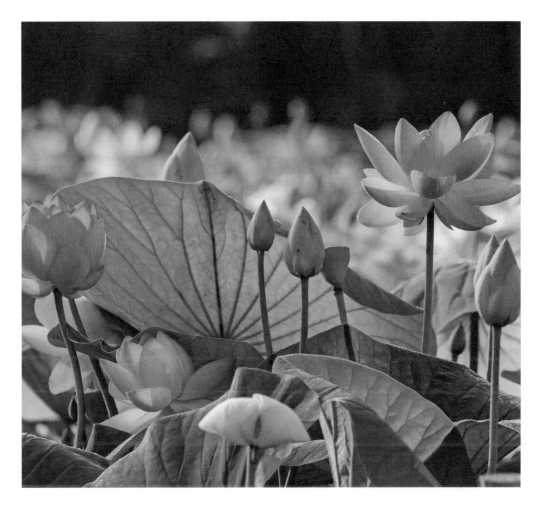

Prepared from the mycelia of a rare fungus (*Xylaria nigripes*), wuling has been used to treat insomnia, anxiety, and depression for 2,000 years.

Mexican calea (*Calea ternifolia* syn. *C. zachatechichi*) is also known as bitter-grass, dream herb, and calea. This plant has been used in Mexico for centuries to induce dreaming sleep. It may increase REM sleep associated with more vivid dreaming—human studies confirm an increase in the frequency, recall, and lucidity of dreams.

Opposite: The sleep-inducing properties of *Lactuca sativa* (lettuce) are contained in the white latex in its stems.
Above: *Nelumbo nucifera* (lotus) induced deep sleep in Odysseus and his men in Greek mythology.

Valeriana officinalis

VALERIAN

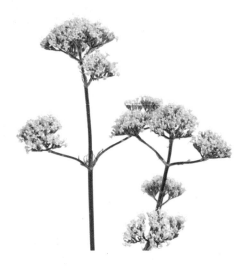

This elegant plant, the roots of which most people consider foul-smelling, is renowned as a traditional sedative and sleeping aid. It has become increasingly popular in recent years as science shows how valerian promotes restful sleep and relaxes the central nervous system (and vets have found this works in dogs, too).

ABOUT THE PLANT: A perennial from Europe and north Asia that grows up to 39 inches (1 m), valerian thrives in damp areas and has lance-shaped, segmented leaves, furrowed stems, and small scented white or pinkish flowers. The roots (harvested in autumn) may smell like old socks but the sweet-scented flowers were once used for perfume. An alternative common name, garden heliotrope, reflects the plant's habit of following the path of the sun. *V. officinalis* is most used in Europe, but Mexican *V. mexicana*, Tibetan *V. jutamansii* and Indian valerian *V. wallichii* are also considered active.

HISTORY AND FOLKLORE: Used in magic for protection from evil and nightmares. The name may derive from *valere* (Latin for "healthy") and it was also called all heal in the Middle Ages. As it's attractive to cats and also rats, legend suggests valerian may have been used as well as music to lure away rats in the Pied Piper of Hamelin. Referred to as "phu" by first- and second-century AD physicians Dioscorides and Galen, who, despite its offensive odor, extolled it for curing epilepsy. Known as the "herbal tranquilizer", valerian has been used in many cultures since the sixteenth century as a safe sedative and tranquilizer (for anxiety, stress, panic and as an anticonvulsant) and to help induce sleep (it was used during World War II by civilians in Britain). Often used in herbal medicine in conjunction with other sedative plants such as passionflower and hop.

WHAT SCIENTISTS SAY

In humans: Most studies in Germany and Switzerland since the 1960s have shown valerian enhances sleep and treats insomnia. A meta-analysis from over sixteen controlled clinical trials concludes valerian improves sleep onset, quality, and length, lowers periods of wakefulness, and has few side effects. Bioactive valerian ingredients (valepotriates) were comparable to the antipsychotic drug chlorpromazine and had weaker but significant sedative effect but, unlike chlorpromazine, valerian actually improved coordination. Valerian also clinically helps to relieve insomnia during menopause, nervous tension and restlessness, and withdrawal from benzodiazepine tranquilizers. It calms children during tooth extraction, and reduces agitation in depression and obsessive compulsive behaviors.

In the lab: Valerian's ingredients act in different ways on the brain's calming signal (GABA; benzodiazepine). They enhance the brain's sleep signal (adenosine) and mood-boosting signal (serotonin) and increase slow-wave (consolidates non-REM) sleep. Valerian also decreases spasms, is anticonvulsant, and neuroprotective.

Many controlled trials confirm the sedative value of valerian, and researchers at São Paulo University in Brazil examined its key ingredients (valepotriates 300 mg/day) on poor sleepers with benzodiazepine dependency. Compared to placebo, those on valepotriates were found to have improved slow-wave sleep, deep sleep, and sleep ratings after benzodiazepine withdrawal

KEY INGREDIENTS: A number of valerian chemicals (not present in all types of products) are responsible for the sedative activity: the valepotriates (which break down to the smelly isovaleric acid, which is also sedative); the sesquiterpenes (such as valerenic acid, which is also in hop); flavonoids (such as methylapigenin); and the more recently discovered linerin and antianxiety and neuroprotective hesperidin (also in bitter orange and passionflower). Essential oil contains the calming ingredients alpha-pinene, patchoulol, bornyl acetate, valerianal, and bisabolene—related to bisabolol in chamomile.

HOW TO TAKE IT: The root tea may well be effective but capsules, tablets, and tincture (150 g dried chopped root in 500 ml 40% alcohol agitated daily for two weeks then strained and stored in a dark glass bottle; 5 ml 2 to 3 times daily) are more palatable. In herbal medicine it is recommended to start with a low dose and work up; a dose can vary according to a person's "nervous constitution," allow 2 to 3 weeks for effects, can be used long term. Young fresh leaves are delicious in salads and seventeenth-century British herbalist John Gerard refers to valerian's use in cooking in poorer parts of north England: "No broth or pottage or physicall meats be worth anything if Setewale [old name for valerian] be not there."

SAFETY: Not with other sleep-inducing drugs, alcohol, or anesthetics as combined actions are stronger and potentially hazardous. Not usually advisable in depression, but can be used with St John's wort. Not usually recommended in pregnancy. Rare liver toxicity reported probably due to adulteration of product. Taking valerian occasionally provokes individual reactions such as headaches. One study suggests valerian does not affect driving simulator performance. Listed in British and US pharmacopoeias and has UK Traditional Herbal Medicine registration for sleep. Not to be confused with the highly poisonous hemlock, looking similar, with a malodorous root.

Valerian nightcap

A nip (1 teaspoon) of brandy infused with valerian root and other sleep-inducing plants such wild lettuce, hop, passionflower and chamomile flowers makes a soothing nightcap.

Plants in the bedroom

Reasons to keep plants in the bedroom are numerous. Some purify the air, for example mother-in-law's tongue (*Sansevieria trifasciata*), English ivy (*Hedera helix*), aloe, and ferns. Or you might choose a spider plant (*Chlorophytum comosum*), which mops up formaldehyde in the atmosphere.

Also try a few aromatic, sleep-inducing plants such as lavender, chamomile, valerian, or jasmine which, even if they don't emit their scents so strongly at night, will have added their scent to the room during the day.

Some people worry about keeping plants in the room you sleep in because of the carbon dioxide they produce, but some plants produce oxygen at night. Whichever species you choose, a few plants will emit a lot less carbon dioxide than a partner!

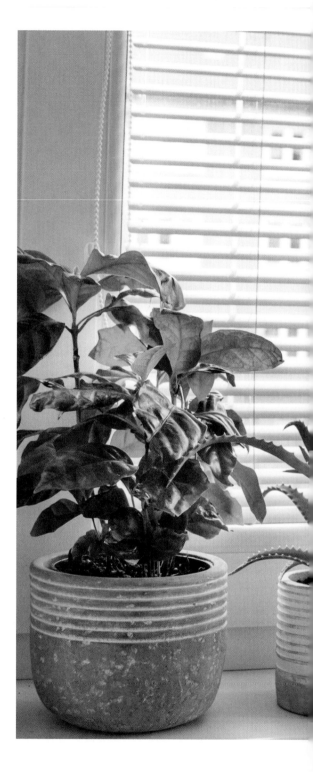

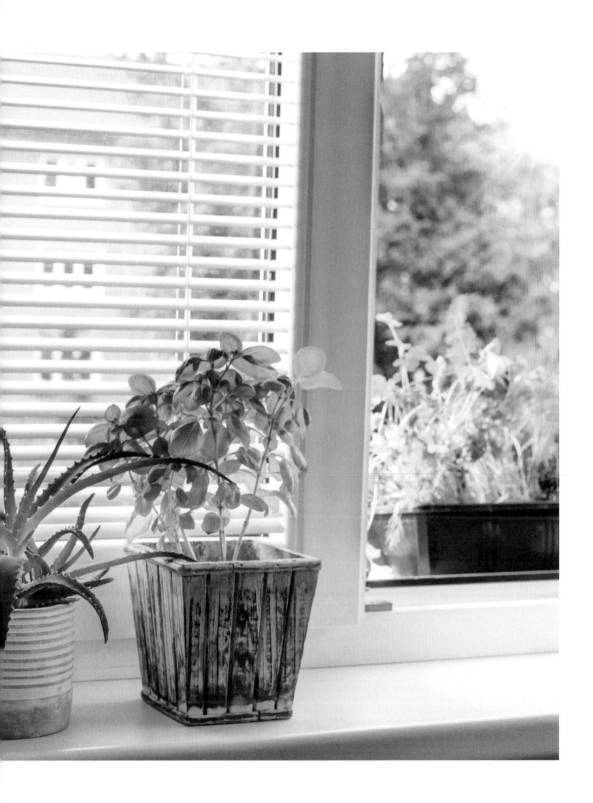

Humulus lupulus

HOP

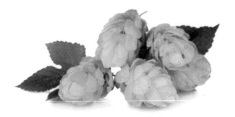

The bitter taste of hop is well known to beer drinkers so it's no surprise that this soporific plant has a marked relaxing and tranquilizing effect on the central nervous system and is used extensively (often in combination with valerian) for insomnia.

ABOUT THE PLANT: Native to Europe, western Asia, and North America, and grown commercially all over Europe, this is a vigorous climber that reaches great heights. It has coarse-toothed, heart-shaped leaves and distinctive cone-like greenish flowers that are gathered when fully ripe. Hop is in the same family as cannabis (Cannabaceae), which is also sleep inducing.

HISTORY AND FOLKLORE: The Romans ate the young shoots in spring in the same way as we eat asparagus (and there is growing demand for the young shoots today). Named *lupulus* from Latin *lupus* (wolf), because it strangles any plant it climbs up, as the wolf does a sheep. The English name "hop" comes from the Anglo-Saxon *hoppan* (to climb). Described by the British Parliament as "a wicked weed" in the sixteenth century, hop is added to beer as a preservative and used today for flavoring in a plethora of local beers made with a variety of other herbs. In herbal medicine it is used in a

variety of ways: as a hypnotic and sedative for insomnia and other sleep disorders, and for restlessness, tension, excitability, attention-deficit hyperactivity disorder (ADHD), and spasms. According to Andrew Chevallier, "A sachet placed inside a bed pillow releases an aroma that calms the mind."

WHAT SCIENTISTS SAY

In humans: Most controlled studies of hop are in combination with valerian (*Valeriana officinalis*). A meta-analysis concluded this combination is effective for sleep and a multicenter study concluded it is as effective as antihistamines for mild insomnia. A hop-valerian combination is also effective in a single dose, more so than valerian alone, and equal to a benzodiazepine for temporary insomnia. A combination of hop, valerian and passionflower was found to be as safe and as effective as the sedative Zolpidem. Hop in combination with lavender oil, lemon balm, and oat altered electrical brain activity consistent with a state of relaxation. As capsules in a controlled trial, hop decreases depression and stress scores; as a nonalcoholic beer, it decreases the time taken to fall asleep in nurses and students, and decreases anxiety. Several studies show benefits for menopausal symptoms, which can disturb sleep.

In the lab: Hop depresses the central nervous system, increasing the calming neurotransmitter (GABA). It also affects brain sleep signals such as melatonin and adenosine and the serotonin (mood-boosting) transmitter. In lab models hop increases pentobarbital sleep enhancement and together with valerian reduces caffeine-induced arousal, has analgesic effects, and is antispasmodic.

KEY INGREDIENTS: A bitter resin called lupulin (that oozes out of glands in the flowers and dries to a yellowish powder), isovaleric acid (a sedative ingredient also in valerian), flavonoids, essential oil containing humulene (also present in cannabis). Contains low amounts of a potent phytoestrogen (8-prenylnaringenin) and xanthohumol, which is antioxidant.

HOW TO TAKE IT: Tea of 2 to 3 g dried (4 to 6 g fresh) flowers per 240 ml 3 times daily (with one cup taken at night) sweetened with honey as it is bitter. Also taken as a tincture, capsules, tablets, and enjoy young shoots blanched as a fresh vegetable.

SAFETY: Some suggest avoiding in depression. Caution in hormone-sensitive cancers and conditions.

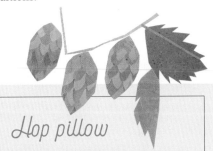

Hop pillow

Hop is a beautiful plant to grow so use fresh flowers if you have them at hand or alternatively buy them dried. With right sides together, machine sew three sides of a folded rectangle of muslin. Turn right side out, fill with hop flowers and machine sew the fourth side. Use embroidery stitches to decorate with hop and lavender. Dab with a few drops of hops, and or lavender essential oil before use.

Chamaemelum nobile syn. *Anthemis nobilis*, *Chamomilla recutita* syn. *Matricaria recutita*

CHAMOMILE

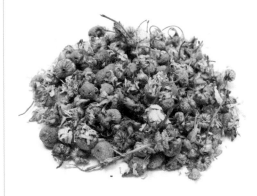

Chamomile is one of the oldest known medicinal plants and the most popular herbal tea to help sleep and relieve anxiety (an estimated 1 million cups are consumed every day). With diverse mind and body benefits, its distinctive apple-like scented oil is in part responsible for its sedative and calming actions.

ABOUT THE PLANT: Both species grow wild on poor soil in sun in Europe and are cultivated widely. Both are self-seeding annuals or biennials in the daisy family. German or blue chamomile (*Chamomilla recutita*) grows to 2 feet (60 cm) with daisy-like white and yellow flowers. Roman or common chamomile, *Chamaemelum nobile*, also called ground or earth apple, is creeping and nonflowering, and is propagated by division. The cultivar Treneague is suitable for preparing lawns: "the more it is trodden on, the faster it grows," wrote Shakespeare in *Henry IV*. Both species thrive in pots. Easily confused with similar-looking plants, chamomile is said to heal and help other plants to grow.

HISTORY AND FOLKLORE: Both species have been used in a similar way. Used as incense by the Romans, though not cultivated in Rome until the sixteenth century. The famous seventeenth-century English herbalist John Parkinson said, "Camomil is put to divers and sundry uses, both for pleasure and profit, both for the sick and the sound, in bathing to comfort and strengthen the sound and to ease pains in the diseased." In Europe and the Middle East, chamomile is widely used in herbal medicine and aromatherapy as a sedative (especially in children) to promote sleep, to calm and relieve anxiety, and as a relaxant for restlessness and irritability. Also used to relieve headaches, migraines, arthritis, menstrual and menopausal problems—all linked to disturbed sleep.

WHAT SCIENTISTS SAY

In humans: A controlled trial shows chamomile significantly improves daytime function in insomniacs. In preliminary trials, chamomile tea during cardiac catheterization induces deep sleep in ten out of twelve patients. The tea also reduces sleep problems and depression in postnatal women compared to those not taking it (and when they stopped drinking it so did their improved sleep). Further clinical studies confirm the sleep-inducing traditional use of chamomile essential oil in aromatherapy. Inhaling the essential oil produces a sedative effect in volunteers and in combination with lavender and neroli, chamomile inhalation improves sleep and anxiety in coronary care patients.

Relieving anxiety is closely linked to a good night's sleep and in controlled trials chamomile is comparable to conventional drugs effective for moderate to severe anxiety. Fifty-seven people with mild anxiety taking one chamomile capsule a day for two weeks had a greater reduction in anxiety than the placebo and in a separate controlled study chamomile showed antidepressive effects. Adults with attention-deficit hyperactivity disorder (ADHD) taking chamomile for four weeks had improved hyperactivity, inattention, and irritability scores. Chamomile also reduces hot flushes, is anticonvulsant (childhood) and analgesic (in teething, earache, osteoporosis) and, in a controlled trial, as effective as the drug diclofenac for knee osteoarthritis). A population study (not necessarily cause

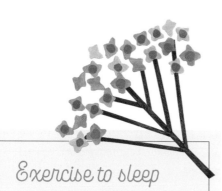

Exercise to sleep

It is hard to overstate the benefits of vigorous bursts of daytime exercise, which has also been shown to promote nighttime sleep. So just choose your spot, beside the bed or a container of valerian flowers or perhaps a chamomile lawn, and practise tai chi or yoga. If plants are not on hand, sprinkle essential oil of valerian (oil made from plant is better than root) or chamomile over your outdoor yoga spot. Then, last thing at night, to help relaxation and sleep, focus on breathing and stretching every muscle in turn when lying in bed.

and effect) in 2015 suggests chamomile consumption in 1,677 people over the age of 65 years is protective against mortality in older women but not men.

In the lab: Both plant extracts and ingredients apigenin, chrysin, and pinenes act on brain calming (GABA) signals, are central nervous system (CNS) depressant, and increase sleep latency. Effect is benzodiazepine-like, although other brain signals are involved (such as noradrenaline and the enzyme monoamine oxidase). When the dose is increased ten-fold the antianxiety effects are combined with the mild sedation and the inhaled essential oil decreases stress reaction in lab models. No detrimental effect on memory shown. Chamomile is also antispasmodic, analgesic, anti-inflammatory and antioxidant (bisabolol and chamazulene in lab tests).

KEY INGREDIENTS: Flavonoids (such as apigenin, luteolin, chrysin), tannins, and coumarins. The essential oil contains farnesene, bisabolol, and chamazulene (formed from matricine during distillation) in German chamomile; and iso-butyl, methylbutyl angelates, and pinenes in Roman chamomile.

HOW TO TAKE IT: Tea 2 to 3 g fresh (4 to 6 g dried) flower heads or leaves per 240 ml water 3 times daily (German tastes best but Roman is better for nausea and stomach cramp) with honey if required to sweeten. Tincture and capsules also used, and the essential oils for aromatherapy use.

SAFETY: Safe, though some caution Roman, in pregnancy. No restrictions on long-term use. Roman chamomile may cause rare contact dermatitis in the susceptible.

Ziziphus jujuba var. *spinosa*

JUJUBE OR SUAN ZAO REN

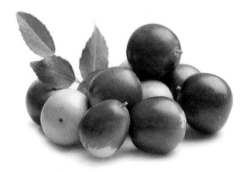

This traditional Chinese medicine has a reputation for treating disturbed dreams. It comes with a promising evidence base as a sedative for insomnia and for treating anxiety.

ABOUT THE PLANT: Also known as spina or sour date seed, this is a thorny, drought-resistant shrub. Growing in China, Europe, and Australia, it reaches 10 feet (3 m) and has small yellow-green flower clusters that turn into a purple-black, wrinkled, date-like fruit. There are forty species of *Ziziphus* and others (such as *Z. jujube* var. *inermis*) are used for different indications in Chinese medicine.

HISTORY AND FOLKLORE: Known as the Chinese date, this "fruit of life" has long been widely consumed for its nutritional benefits in China. Also known as *annab* in Iran, *ber* in India and *pomme surette* in French, its sweet, edible fruit is dried, and legend has it that it causes teenagers to fall in love. As a traditional Chinese medicine, jujube been used as a sedative for thousands of years, and more recently in other countries. It is increasingly used in Europe to combat insomnia and "dream-disturbed sleep." It's the second most common plant medicine for insomnia in Taiwan. Also used in herbal medicine today to calm, for anxiety, irritability, and palpitations.

WHAT SCIENTISTS SAY

In humans: The Chinese herbal medicine formulation (zao ren tang), which contains jujube, in combination with smaller amounts of five other sedative plants, significantly increased sleep quality and daytime function, without side effects, in a number of pilot clinical trials. In one controlled trial, zao ren tang improved sleep quality and total time asleep in methadone-maintained patients who had sleep problems.

In the lab: The plant and its saponins, flavonoids, and alkaloids (in seed and fruit) are sedative, enhance barbiturate-induced hypnotic effects, and reduce anxiety in several models. It enhances calming (GABA) and sleep (histamine) brain signals and also works at mood-boosting (serotonin) and excitatory (glutamate) signals. Jujube also has anticonvulsant, neuroprotective, and memory-enhancing capacity effect, as well as antiaging and pain-relieving effects.

KEY INGREDIENTS: Saponins (soapy constituents) such as jujubosides, flavonoids (such as spinosin), and alkaloids (such as sanjoinine), are sedative and reduce anxiety. Also contains fatty acids such as steric, linoleic, oleic.

HOW TO TAKE IT: Eat the delicious fresh or dried fruits (up to 50 g dried fruit daily). Seeds and fruit can also be taken as tea, tincture, wine, syrup, pastes, or added to puddings and cakes.

SAFETY: Caution with SSRI (selective serotonin reuptake inhibitor) antidepressants. Not in pregnancy (due to traditional antifertility reputation).

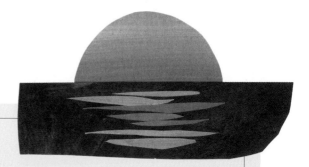

Salute to the setting sun

Yoga is good for sleep. Along with other meditative movements, daily "salutes to the sun" or "asanas" at sunset will, according to studies, promote nighttime relaxation. In a 2016 review of controlled trials on tai chi, qi gong, and yoga, the psychology department at Guang'an hospital in Beijing found that in seventeen high-quality clinical trials, meditative movement was beneficial on a range of sleep measures. And doing salutes as the sun sets is best, since sunlight increases vitamin D and studies show higher vitamin D is associated with increased sleep.

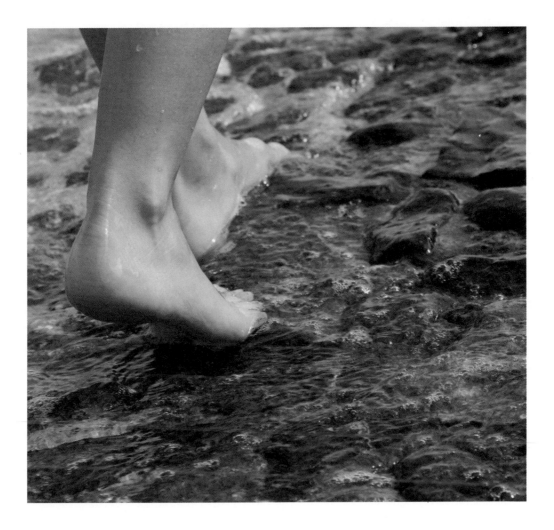

Sleep-promoting foot massage

Walk around in bare feet to massage the acupuncture points that promote sleep. Several pilot clinical studies, and one controlled trial, show reflexology improves sleep. In one pilot trial a particular type of Chinese reflexology (shujing massage) actually performed better than a benzodiazepine (estazolam) in increasing sleep, though more research is needed. Sprinkle drops of essential oil or strew leaves of lemon balm and flowers of lavender, chamomile, chrysanthemum, and passionflower where you walk regularly, either on a floor inside or a lawn outside, to capture some of the aromatics that work on the brain to induce sleep.

Prunus cerasus syn. *Cerasus vulgaris*

TART CHERRY

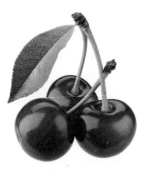

Tart cherry is one of the few natural sources of our brain's essential sleep signal melatonin. Clinical trials show it increases the duration and the quality of sleep.

ABOUT THE PLANT: Tart, wild, sour, or morello cherry trees can grow to 40 feet (12 m). They are native to Europe and Southeast Asia and cultivated widely. Deciduous, with serrated leaves and pinkish-white flowers, they have large, dark red, acid fruits. There are more than 270 varieties of tart cherry, a few of them commercially important such as Montmorency, Richmond, and English Morello.

HISTORY AND FOLKLORE: In Scottish Highland folklore, if one encountered a sour cherry it was auspicious. Commonly used in Portugal medicinally in the fifteenth century, it forms the basis of their popular liqueur *ginjinha*. Listed in nineteenth- and twentieth-century US pharmacopoeias as a sedative, proving both Native Americans and early settlers correct. In herbal medicine it's used as a central nervous system sedative in convalescence, heart palpitations, and nervous diseases.

WHAT SCIENTISTS SAY

In humans: Tart cherry increases melatonin and the duration and quality of sleep in controlled studies. In a number of other clinical studies, it raises mood, increases serotonin (the brain's mood-boosting signal), decreases stress (lowering the stress hormone cortisol), and is a key antioxidant. In a controlled study, wild cherry improved vascular function (such as lowering blood pressure, which is associated with sleep) in 27 volunteers. It also relieved pain in several controlled trials.

In two controlled studies with volunteers, carried out at Northumbria University in England and Extremadura University in Spain, drinking tart cherry juice increased melatonin and was beneficial in improving the total time asleep and the quality of sleep in men and women, young and old.

In the lab: There are only a few studies to date. It improves working memory and is antioxidant and anti-inflammatory.

KEY INGREDIENTS: Melatonin, tryptophan, and serotonin. Rich in anthocyanins, responsible for red/purple pigments (such as asterin and prunetin) that are anti-inflammatory, antioxidant, and reduce cholesterol.

HOW TO TAKE IT: Tart cherries are eaten as a food, or drunk as a juice; up to 220 g juiced taken 2 times daily is said to improve sleep. Also take as a tincture.

SAFETY: Treat as a foodstuff. No contraindications or side effects known.

Tart cherry lemonade

1 pound (450 g) pitted fresh cherries
(or thawed if frozen)
1 cup (200 g) granulated sugar
1 scant cup (225 ml) water
Juice of 4 lemons

To Serve:
Ice cubes
I quart (1 L) sparkling water
Fresh cherries to garnish

For the syrup, simmer the cherries, granulated sugar, water, and lemon juice in a medium saucepan over medium heat until the cherries are broken down and juicy and the liquid is syrupy, about 30 minutes.

Strain the syrup through a fine mesh sieve. Allow the syrup to cool.

Add ice cubes, ½ cup (125 ml) cherry syrup and the sparkling water to a large pitcher and stir to combine.

Divide the lemonade among glasses. Garnish with fresh cherries and valerian leaves.

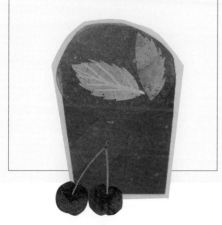

Eschscholzia californica

CALIFORNIA POPPY

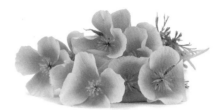

This poppy brightens gardens around the world with its orange and yellow flowers, and new research is exploring the science behind its strong reputation in herbal medicine as a safe and gentle sedative plant.

ABOUT THE PLANT: Native to the United States and growing wild across California and other parts of North America as well as South America and France, this poppy is cultivated throughout the world. An annual or perennial growing to 2 feet (60 cm), it has fine deep-cut leaves and bright orange or yellow flowers that close at sunset. Although related to the opium poppy, it has very different effects and is not narcotic. Aerial parts are collected when flowering.

HISTORY AND FOLKLORE: Traditionally used to induce sleep by Native Americans and rural populations of California by speeding up onset and improving the duration of sleep. Also used in herbal medicine for relieving pain (such as toothache and colic) and for treating overexcitability and sleeplessness in children (antispasmodic). Its safe sedative, anti-anxiety and analgesic, effects mean this plant medicine is sold in pharmacies in many countries. The flowers, high in carotenoids, are slightly sweet when chewed and their rich pollen is used as body paint.

WHAT SCIENTISTS SAY

In humans: When taken with hawthorn (*Crataegus ripidophylla* syn. *C. oxyacantha*) and magnesium in a controlled trial, the California poppy proved safe and more effective than placebo in treating anxiety disorder—important for a good night's sleep. In combination with *Corydalis cava* (both have active isoquinoline alkaloids), two trials show normalization of disturbed sleep behaviors.

In the lab: It is sedative and prolongs sleep, lowers motor activity (antispasmodic), is neuroprotective and antidepressant in lab models. This plant affects the brain's calming (GABA) and mood-boosting (serotonin) signals and also prevents the breakdown of other amine signals like dopamine (via monoamine oxidase) and synthesis of adrenaline (the alert, fight or flight signal.)

KEY INGREDIENTS: The latex is sedative and painkilling. Contains (isoquinalone) alkaloids similar to opium poppy, and others such as californidine, sanguinarine, and eschscholtzine which are much less narcotic than alkaloids such as morphine and codeine. Also contains flavonoid glycosides (such as rutin), carotenoids, and an essential oil.

HOW TO TAKE IT: Tea of aerial parts 1 to 2 gm in 240 ml water at night, with honey as it's bitter. Capsules and tincture also used.

SAFETY: Commonly prescribed for children (also for nocturnal enuresis). Nonaddictive. May interact with drugs metabolized by cytochrome P450s. Not in glaucoma or with MAOIs, tranquilizers or other CNS depressants. Do not mistake for opium poppy (*Papaver somniferum*). Avoid in pregnancy and breastfeeding.

Verbena officinalis

VERVAIN

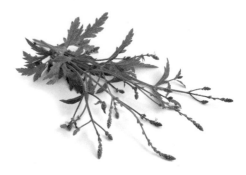

This traditional sedative is a gentle aid to those suffering from stress and exhaustion. Used in herbal medicine as a restorative tonic, it is still short of scientific research.

ABOUT THE PLANT: Growing wild through most of Europe, North Africa, Japan, and China, vervain likes the sun and is easily cultivated in pots. A hairy, branching, self-seeding perennial, it has slim wand-like angular stems up to 3 feet (90 cm) with toothed three-lobed greenish-grey leaves. It has sparse but attractive small lilac flowers, and aerial parts are harvested just before flowers open.

HISTORY AND FOLKLORE: In the first century Dioscorides called vervain the sacred herb; it was also called herba sacra (priests used it for sacrifices) and herb of the cross as it was said to have been used to stem the wounds of Christ. Folklore credits it with magical and aphrodisiacal properties. It was popular as a panacea with the druids and was regarded as a sacred plant in ancient Rome. Carried in the Middle Ages to bring good luck and worn around the neck against headaches, it was used in the herbal medicine of Europe and China as a mild sedative and nervine (calming), and as a tonic and strengthener. Traditionally used for its parasympathetic action, vervain relieves tension, anxiety, long-term stress and exhaustion. Known as *ma bian cao*, it is used (with other herbs) in traditional Chinese medicine for headaches and migraines, particularly associated with the menstrual cycle.

WHAT SCIENTISTS SAY

In humans: The only controlled clinical multicenter trial was for gingivitis, not sleep. Importantly for a first trial, there were no side effects.

In the lab: Vervain is sedative, antianxiety, and anticonvulsant in several lab models. Neuroprotective (protects against neuronal loss and is antioxidant), its ingredient cornin increases the formation of new blood vessels after stroke. Also anti-inflammatory and analgesic.

KEY INGREDIENTS: Alkaloids, mucilage, tannins, essential oil, bitter glycosides such as verbenalin and cornin. Also contains flavonoids such as apigenin and luteolin (the major flavonoid in calming lemon balm).

HOW TO TAKE IT: A tea made from 4 to 6 g fresh or 2 to 3 g dried aerial parts per 240 ml water 3 times daily. Tincture also used.

SAFETY: Do not exceed stated dose, overdose may cause vomiting (it's also used to stimulate digestion and its constituent verbenalin is a mild purgative). Not in pregnancy as it stimulates the uterus.

Take control of your dreams

Pleasant dreams and lucid dreaming (where the dreamer is asleep but aware and able to control their dream) are also enhanced by some plants. Actively inducing lucid dreaming is being researched for its ability to relieve anxiety and post-traumatic stress disorder. People report being more in control of their lives when more in control of their dreams. In folklore, mugwort and vervain promote lucid dreaming (people come back every year to Dilston Physic Garden to buy mugwort to help with sleep and dreaming). For anyone suffering from repeated nightmares, there are hosts of plants used traditionally for relief—valerian, hyacinth, cedar, jasmine, marjoram, mullein, garlic, and thyme—but so far the science is lacking.

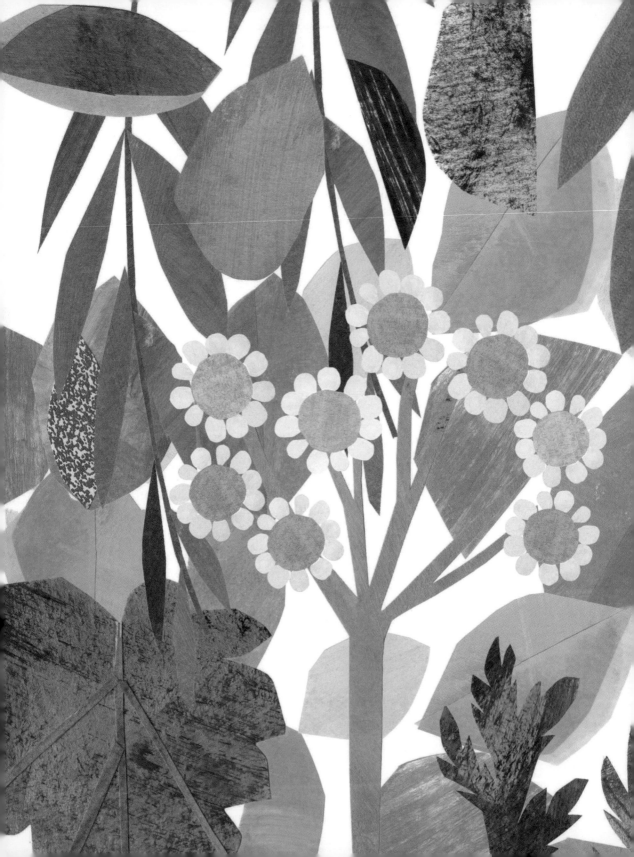

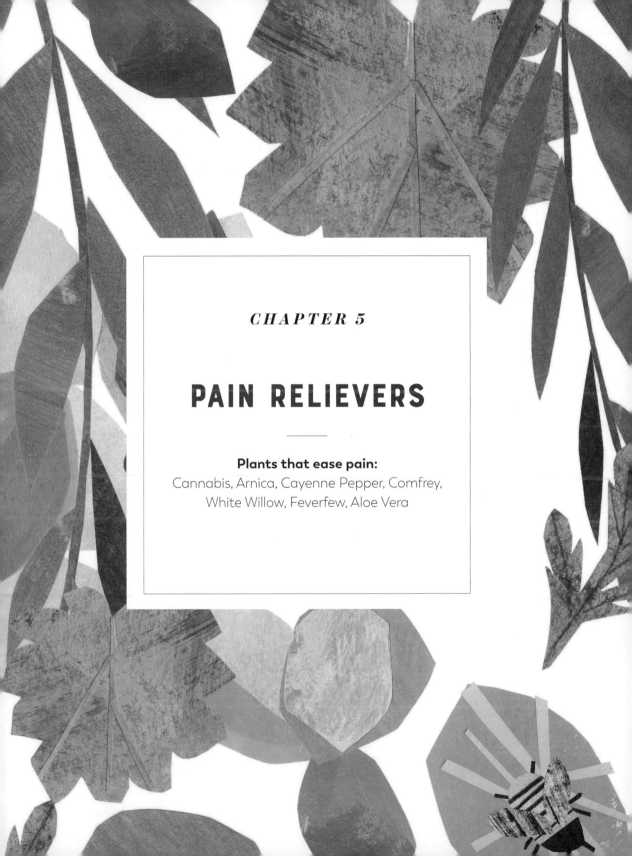

CHAPTER 5

PAIN RELIEVERS

———

Plants that ease pain:
Cannabis, Arnica, Cayenne Pepper, Comfrey,
White Willow, Feverfew, Aloe Vera

Why would plants have a role in pain relief? Surely it can't be to their biological advantage to relieve pain in animals, but the opium poppy, with its silken flowers and seed pods shaped like incense censers are a magnetic draw for both insects and mammals alike. Known first as an analgesic (pain-relieving) plant, the opium poppy's active ingredient morphine paved the way to discovery of the brain's own endorphin-based pain-control system. To explore this and the contribution of other less well-known but safer plants for pain relief, let's look at the mechanisms involved in pain.

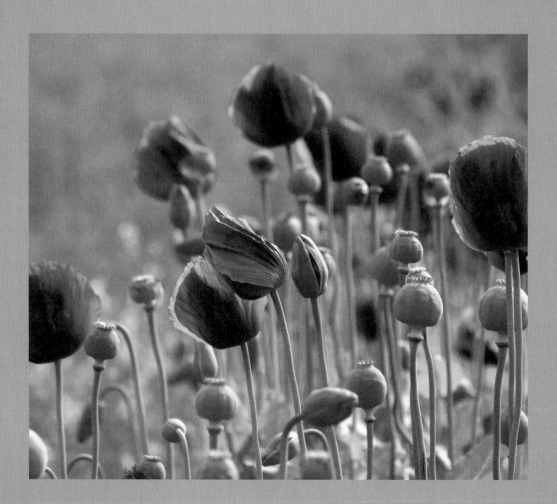

PUTTING PAINKILLERS IN BOXES

Pain perception involves physical sensations and reactions and, for cognitive creatures such as ourselves, is connected to processes of conscious awareness and emotion. Pain is perceived and interpreted within the brain with signals that control attention (such as our memory signal acetylcholine) or pleasure (such as dopamine, serotonin, and our endogenous cannabinoids). Other signals, for example GABA and substance P and others that help to reduce the inflammatory reaction are involved, too.

Plant painkillers are of two types—those that act locally in the body and those that act centrally in the brain. Central pain relievers use signals such as the endorphins while local ones concentrate on the cascade of inflammatory mediators generated by the immune system—mediators such as cytokines, that in turn affect white blood cells and vascular responses such as prostaglandin release (which itself can cause pain). Plants take a central role on this stage because so many contain anti-inflammatory ingredients like the polyphenols. Some well-known anti-inflammatory chemicals from plants are colchicine (a drug from autumn crocus, used to treat gout), resveratrol (in grapes and cocoa), epigallocatechin-3-gallate or EGCG (in green tea) and quercetin (found in brightly colored fruits and vegetables). Any single plant can contain more than one active ingredient, and each may act synergistically on different inflammatory mediators. The most famous anti-inflammatory plant is the white willow (*Salix alba*)—and aspirin, derived from its bark, is still the world's most widely used drug.

PAIN MANAGEMENT

Potent painkillers can be addictive and risk lives. In 2017, Canada and the USA reported record numbers of deaths from addictive opioid prescription painkillers and illegal opioids. Severe inflammatory and neuropathic (nerve damage) pain is usually treated with opioids such as codeine, tramadol, and morphine, which act on opiate receptors in the brain, the molecules that bind the body's natural pain-killing endorphins and enkephalins.

DIFFERENT TYPES OF OPIATE RECEPTORS

Of the three molecules (receptors) that bind opiates, just one μ (called mu) is implicated in addiction. Some plants, including divine sage (*Salvia divinorum*), produce opiate-like chemicals that act on other opiate receptors (such as kappa) and are analgesic but nonaddictive.

Anti-inflammatory drugs do not fall into the high-risk opiate category because they work in different ways. Mild pain (due to external or internal tissue damage) can be managed by analgesics such as paracetamol and nonsteroidal anti-inflammatory drugs (NSAIDs)

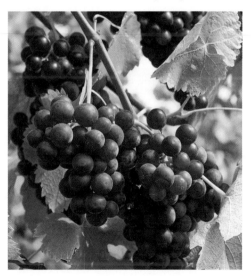

Opposite: The discovery of morphine in opium poppy led to greater understanding of the brain's pain-control system.
Above: *Vitis vinifera* (grape) contains the anti-inflammatory resveratrol.

such as aspirin and ibuprofen, which block prostaglandins released by the body at tissue damage that trigger inflammation and pain. But these are not risk free, because intestinal bleeding is a potentially serious side effect (prostaglandins help to protect the lining of the gut).

PLANTS FOR PAIN

We've chosen for this chapter seven key plants for pain listed in order of scientific backing from greatest to least. Here are some previews of them, and other pain-relieving plants, in no particular order. Arnica, an anti-inflammatory plant medicine (not the homeopathic product), is a leading pain balm. According to the Cochrane review, it works as well as ibuprofen, but without triggering side effects such as heartburn. Then there are the cannabis cannabinoids that relieve pain by acting on the body and brain's own cannabinoid signals like anandamides (which are related to prostaglandins and are named after the Sanskrit word *ananda*, meaning bliss or happiness). Salicin, found in willow bark and meadowsweet (*Filipendula ulmaria*), like its derivative aspirin, blocks prostaglandins that cause pain and swelling, but willow bark does not cause internal bleeding because salicin in willow bark is absorbed in the duodenum rather than the stomach. Feverfew (*Tanacetum parthenium*) contains perthenolide that stops vasodilation involved in migraine, while analgesic chile pepper (capsaicin) affects another signal that controls pain.

PAIN AS A RESEARCH TOPIC

One brain transmitter at the center of much of our research is the memory signal acetylcholine, but it does more than help memory and attention. Depending on where it acts within the body, it controls movement,

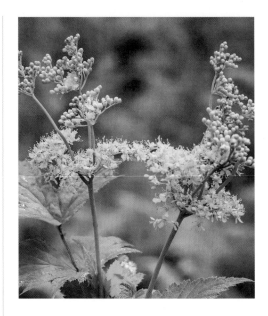

dreaming, pain perception, and may even be a key component of consciousness itself. Plasters of *Atropa belladonna*, which contains a chemical that blocks acetylcholine, are used today to ease local pain. Our research at Newcastle University found that people with dementia who have hallucinations have less acetylcholine, but at the same time others were discovering that people with the Alzheimer's form of dementia experience less pain. We didn't take the idea of reduced pain being due to the loss of acetylcholine further, but we were asked to discuss medicinal plants at a public meeting where people wanted to know more about the link between plants and pain relief. It was then we discovered scientific studies supporting the use of plants for pain that extended way beyond the willow tree or the opium poppy, so we established a "Plants for Pain" area at Dilston Physic Garden.

Above: *Filipendula ulmaria* (meadowsweet) contains salicin that blocks prostaglandins that cause pain.
Opposite: Capsaicin, the active ingredient in chile pepper is used in mainstream medicine for topical pain relief.

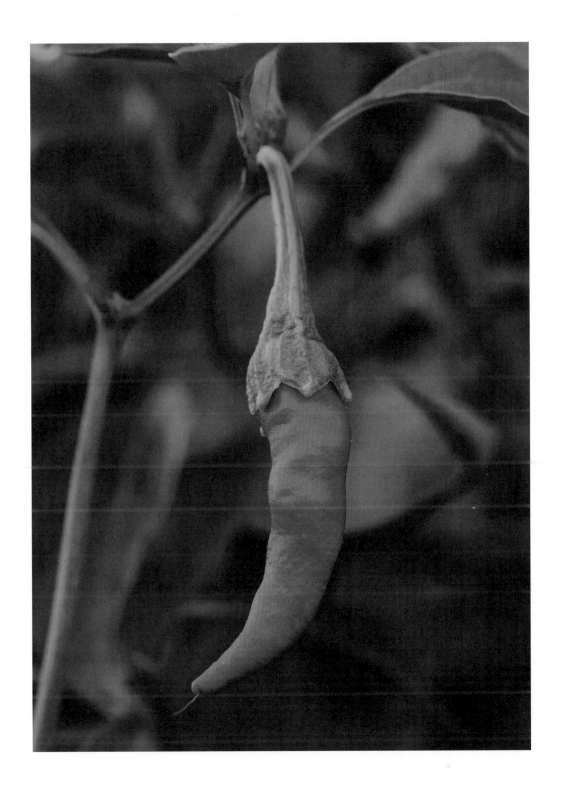

INFLAMMATION AND THE BRAIN

Chronic inflammation of the brain—the organ most confined by space, with little room to accommodate any swelling, and without any sense of local pain to act as a warning—is being billed as a core mechanism involved in depression and dementia. It's little surprise that for a solution people turn to plants, which are almost universally anti-inflammatory.

A TROPICAL PAIN BALM

Kratom (*Mitragyna speciose*), a member of the coffee family native to Thailand, has been used for hundreds of years as a leaf tea in Southeast Asia, taken for fatigue and pain relief and in social and religious functions. Its use for pain has become global and hundreds of thousands of people in the US now take it medicinally. At low doses it gives an energy hit like caffeine,

while at higher doses it's pain relieving (acting like an opiate even though it's not one). A team at the psychiatry department of the University of Rochester in New York studied patients' experiences with kratom. They concluded that not only was it pain relieving and helped people who were quitting drugs like opiates, but it also enhanced relaxation, well-being, empathy and sociability. However, a minority experienced side effects such as nausea, dizziness, and sweats. Some studies indicate regular use can be associated with dependency (certain constituents do involve the μ opioid receptor), although without long-term side effects or social impairment. Extracts contain alkaloids (such as 7-hydroxymitragynine), judged to be "a

Opposite: *Equisetum arvense* (horsetail) is a traditional pain reliever and wound healer.
Below: *Mitragyna speciosa* (kratom)has been taken for pain relief in Southeast Asia for hundreds of years.

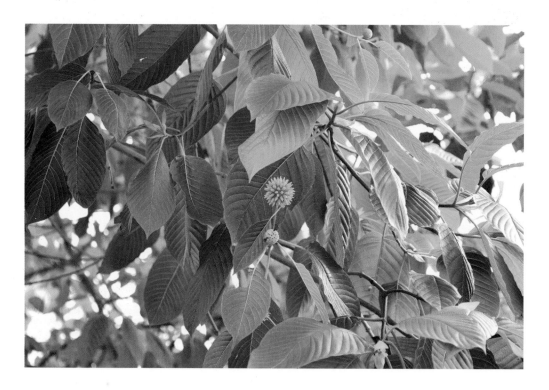

YOUR BRAIN ON PLANTS

13-fold greater opioid (μ receptor) agonist than morphine." However, it seems the whole plant extract is better than the isolated alkaloids, and it may also deserve application in topical pain relief. More study on safety and effects on broader populations is required.

PLANTS WITH SOME SCIENTIFIC BACKING

Many plants are being researched as painkillers including plantain, chaste tree, wintergreen, and camphor. Meadowsweet (*Filipendula ulmaria*), used in Europe to reduce fever and rheumatic pain, and also a great-tasting digestive (4 to 6 g fresh or 2 to 3 g dried plant per 225 ml hot water 3 times daily), reduces inflammation in lab studies. The woody vine *Mandevilla velutina* and Brazilian tree *Protium kleinii* have also been shown in the lab to reduce inflammation and pain.

Horsetail (*Equisetum arvense*), a primitive plant native to northern Asia, North Africa, the Americas, and Europe, traditionally used for pain and wound healing, applied topically promoted wound healing and relieved pain following episiotomy. Dill (*Anethum graveolens*), native to Eurasia, was as effective as a conventional anti-inflammatory in treating dysmenorrhea. The statuesque mullein (*Verbascum thapsus*), traditionally used for centuries for topical inflammation, has been shown (in combination with four other plants) as effective as anesthetic drops for middle ear inflammation in children, along with burdock (*Arctium* species) for pain and inflammation in burns and thunder god vine (*Tripterygium wilfordii*) for pain and inflammation in osteoarthritis.

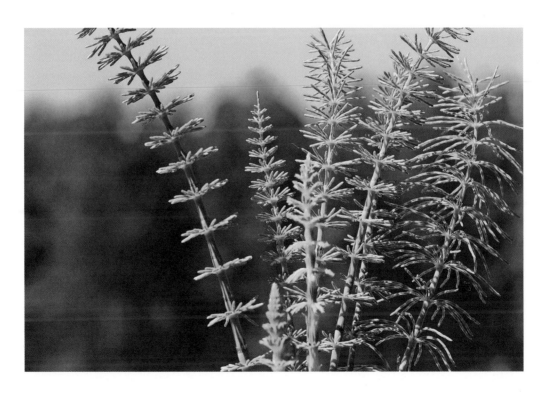

Several clinical trials show that African devil's claw (*Harpagophytum procumbens*) can be used to treat pain and improve movement in osteoarthritis. It has been approved by the German Commission E for "the treatment of degenerative diseases of the musculoskeletal system" and is another example of a plant where the entire plant extract is more effective than isolated parts.

Sesame oil (from *Sesamum indicum*), used in Asia to treat pain and inflammation, is yet another shown by initial trials to be effective in osteoarthritis control—sesamol is thought to be its active ingredient.

The traditional Chinese herbal medicine sanqi (*Panax notoginseng*) and the "king of medicine" in Tibet, myrobalan (*Terminalia chebula*), both have a long history in pain and inflammation control and in initial clinical trials are shown effective for pain relief.

BUTTERBUR TO PREVENT MIGRAINE

Butterbur (*Petasites hybridus*), a flowering plant in the sunflower family that contains the ingredients petasin and isopetasin, has been shown to be antimigraine and anti-inflammatory. In two controlled trials involving migraine sufferers, an extract of butterbur root was judged to be safe and effective in reducing migraine attacks in adults. And in an open label (that is, not placebo-controlled) trial with 108 children (6 to 17 years old) prophylactic (preventative) butterbur reduced the frequency of migraine attacks by at least 50 percent in three quarters of cases. Another controlled study confirmed the benefits of butterbur in childhood migraine. Medical herbalists recommend a root decoction three times daily.

Right: *Petasites hybridus* (butterbur) was judged safe and effective in reducing migraine attacks in adults in two controlled trials.
Far right: Several controlled trials show *Boswellia sacra* (frankincense) effective in pain relief.

Ginger (*Zingiber officinale*) has been shown in several clinical studies to reduce pain and inflammation in osteoarthritis, and in one controlled clinical trial involving 100 migraine sufferers was found to be as effective in reducing headache severity as the orthodox antimigraine drug sumatriptan—and had a better side-effects profile, too.

FRANKINCENSE FOR PAIN

A key anti-inflammatory shown effective for pain relief in several controlled trials. A recent *British Medical Journal* review said "results of all trials indicated that B. serrata extracts were clinically effective." In 2015 a Cochrane review on plant medicines for osteoarthritis came to the same conclusion—although both studies advised that further trials were required. Frankincense is considered a safer anti-inflammatory than corticosteroids for osteoarthritis treatment, and vets find it also works in dogs. Turmeric (*Curcuma longa*) is also a front runner in the plant medicine pain balms race, and a combination of turmeric and frankincense has been shown more effective than the standard dose of celecoxib in osteoarthritis treatment.

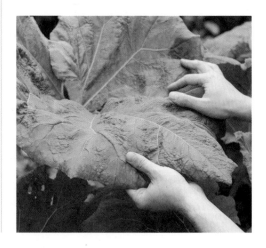

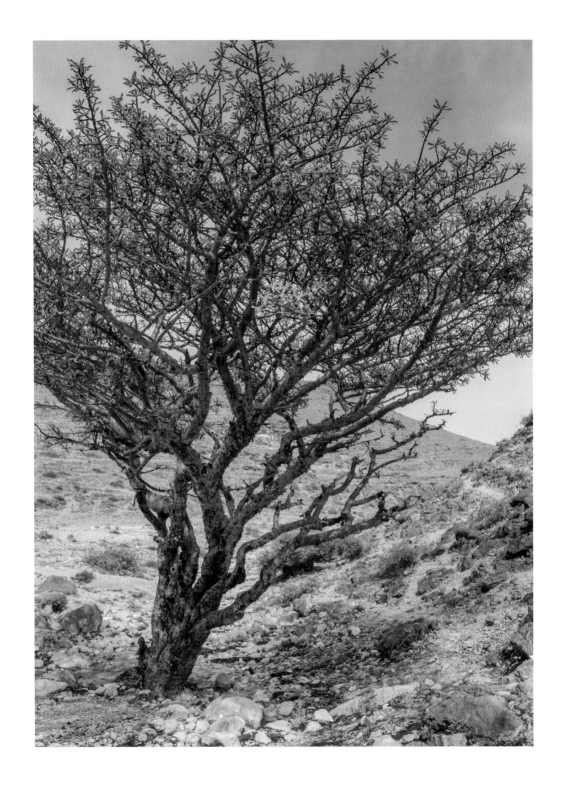

Cannabis sativa syn. *C. indica*

CANNABIS

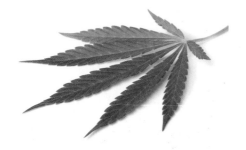

Its recreational reputation overshadows the age-old medicinal use of cannabis, particularly for pain and nausea, now being rediscovered.

ABOUT THE PLANT: Native to northern India, China, and the Caucasus, this annual with long, serrated leaves and creamy flowers reaches 13 feet (4 m) or more in height. It prefers acid soil and grows well in pots. Varieties differ in their content of tetrahydrocannabinol (THC), the mind-altering "high" component, and cannabidiol (CBD), the calming, sedative component.

HISTORY AND FOLKLORE: Cannabis, grown for medicinal, religious, and recreational purposes for thousands of years, was used in ancient Egypt and China and since 800 BC in India, where it's a key plant for pain in Ayurvedic medicine and known as Indian hemp. It was commonly used by European physicians: Queen Victoria took cannabis as an analgesic when it was a standard painkiller for menstrual cramps. In herbal medicine it's used for pain, anxiety, post-traumatic stress, epilepsy, insomnia, arthritis, multiple sclerosis, for nightmares, and in addiction.

WHAT SCIENTISTS SAY

In humans: With over 9,000 references, most trials and reviews are on the individual cannabinoids (such as THC or CBD) rather than the whole plant, so are not reflective of traditional use. Studies are equivocal but controlled trials show that a THC:CBD extract is effective for pain in cancer and in other trials for MS, neuropathic pain, and muscle spasms. A meta-analysis concludes cannabis, as well as synthetically derived cannabinoids such as nabilone and other products such as a THC:CBD spray, is effective in neuropathic and other pain. Some studies show people prefer whole cannabis extract to the synthetic cannabis-derived drugs as it also relieves associated anxiety and depression. Cannabis and the synthetic THC drug dronabinol have been shown to improve ADHD and Tourette's syndrome. Cannabidiol in controlled trials was found safe as a sedative and to reduce psychosis in people with Parkinson's and with schizophrenia, and also improves memory in the latter, without the side effects of standard antipsychotics. It is also antiseizure in controlled trials in children and is being researched for brain trauma.

In the lab: Analgesic (including THC and CBD on their own), sedative, antispasmodic and anti-inflammatory. Acts on brain (and body) signals for endogenous cannabinoids such as anandamine, an arachidonic lipid, and on other brain signals and enzymes (such as monoamine oxidase). Medical research is now focused on cannabidiol, which is anxiolytic, antidepressive, antipsychotic, antiepileptic, neuroprotective, and anticancer but has no "high" effects. CBD also affects the brain's calming signal (GABA) and may stop the anxiety caused by high doses of THC. THC itself is euphoric and sedative and works at spinal and brain levels to relieve pain. THC and opioids may have synergistic analgesic effects. Cannabis and THC decrease the brain's excitatory signal (glutamate), which may be linked to short-term increases in the brain's pleasure signal (dopamine).

KEY INGREDIENTS: Contains about seventy cannabinoids (present in leaves and flower buds) such as cannabidiol and cannabinol, and is the only plant to contain THC, the main mind-altering cannabinoid. Also contains flavonoids, alkaloids, and an essential oil with the anti-inflammatory humulene, the calming linalool, and beta-caryophyllene (which activates cannabinoid signals—C2 receptors) all of which may act synergistically with cannabinoids.

HOW TO TAKE IT: Take as advised by your medical practitioner as regulations regarding medicinal use vary depending on where you live. Medical cannabis is obtained from female flowers and leaves and is standardized to levels of THC and CBD, and administered as tea, tincture, vapor smoking, dermal patches, oral/dermal sprays, or in foodstuffs. Dose can be adjusted to achieve the desired effect.

SAFETY: Of the THC-rich plant (cannabis as opposed to hemp), side effects can include possible short-term cognitive compromise, euphoria, panic or anxiety attacks, as well as others such as dry mouth, reddened eyes, and reduced coordination. Psychosis is cited as a consequence of cannabis abuse but studies have concluded lack of evidence, though it may worsen any pre-existing symptoms. Pure natural and synthetic CBD compounds do not have these disadvantages but may not have the overall therapeutic effect of the plant. Possible

contraindication in cardiovascular disorders and fertility and with other medications since CBD inhibits drug-metabolizing enzymes in the liver. Long-term, recreational cannabis smoking may increase blood pressure.

Legal medicinal use of cannabis varies from country to country and regulations are changing all the time. Seek professional advice from your health care provider.

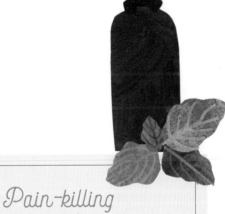

Pain-killing peppermint

Peppermint oil reduced tension headaches in placebo-controlled trials. Ten percent peppermint oil (in ethanol solution) applied topically was as effective as 1000 mg of paracetamol if the treatment was repeated every 15 minutes until the headache had gone. Peppermint blocks serotonin and substance P and increases skin blood flow after local application.

Walking a labyrinth or maze

Moving the body gently is now advised as a better way to help relieve chronic back pain than paracetamol. Walking a labyrinth or maze involves constant turning as you follow a single circuitous path that leads to a central point. If you have enough space in your garden for such a thing, fill the spaces between the path with meadowsweet—the frothy flowers have a delightfully sweet smell.

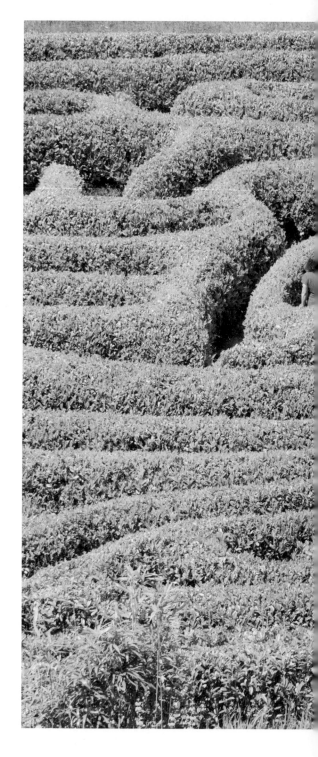

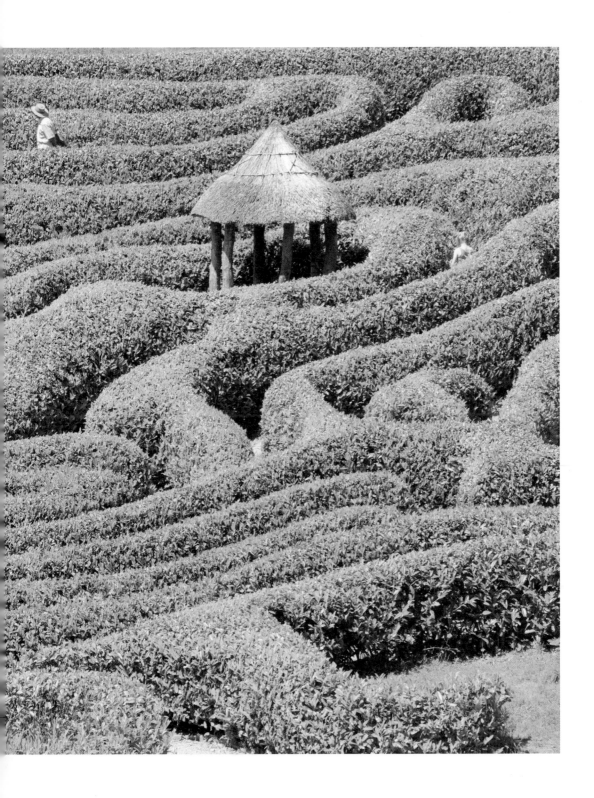

Arnica montana

ARNICA

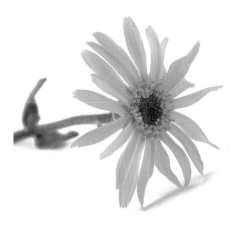

Arnica's use as a plant medicine for relieving pain is well established. Extracts of the plant (not homeopathic products) are verified safe and effective in the topical treatment of osteoarthritis, muscle ache, venous insufficiency, and more.

ABOUT THE PLANT: Native to uplands of central Europe, Siberia, and northern America, this ornamental perennial thrives in wild meadows. It grows to 2 feet (60 cm), with aromatic orange-yellow flowers and veined oval leaves. Plant medicine uses mainly flowers but also root (collected in autumn).

HISTORY AND FOLKLORE: Used for hundreds of years in Europe and known as mountain tobacco (smoking it was once a popular therapeutic practice). The alternative name, leopard's or wolf's bane (it was grown around stock fields to keep out predators) is confusing since the name also belongs to a similar-looking toxic species (*Doronicum orientale*). Arnica tea was once used to relieve chest pain (angina)

and for heart disease and fevers, but the plant is not used internally today. In herbal medicine it is a powerful topical anti-inflammatory and analgesic, stems blood leakage, and is a key wound-healing ointment for sprains, muscle pain, and bruises. Also used for rheumatic pain and for inflamed veins.

WHAT SCIENTISTS SAY

In humans: In controlled clinical trials arnica reduces bruising (better than 1% vitamin K) and postoperative edema, improves wound healing, and relieves muscle pain after extreme exercise. Arnica gel is equipotent to ibuprofen gel for treating hand osteoarthritis—a Cochrane review of topical plant medicines for osteoarthritis concluded that arnica gel improves pain and function as well as nonsteroidal anti-inflammatory drugs. In clinical trials arnica also counters venous insufficiency and is effective for pain relief in knee osteoarthritis, sprains, wounds, bruises, and chilblains. Most trials of the homeopathic product show no significant effect above placebo.

Arnica versus ibuprofen: In a strictly controlled study conducted at a rheumatology clinic in Switzerland, topically applied gel preparations of ibuprofen (5%) or arnica (50% of 1:20 tincture) were equal in their effects for improving pain and hand function after twenty-one days in 204 people.

In the lab: Improves peripheral blood flow and is anti-inflammatory (and antimicrobial) on peripheral application. Arnica stimulates the immune system internally and is a potent anti-inflammatory—its main ingredient dihydrohelanin inhibits inflammatory signals in a similar way to glucocorticoids.

KEY INGREDIENTS: Bitter sesquiterpene lactones (such as helanalin), alkaloids, coumarins (such as scopoletin), tannins, and mucilage/polysaccharides. Flavonoids (such as hispidulin, astragalin and luteolin) and carotenoids (responsible for the color of tincture).

HOW TO TAKE IT: For external use. Flowers and roots used to make gels, lotions, oils, and compresses to 50% concentration (can also use diluted essential oil). Tincture of flowers or root also applied in a compress or added to footbaths.

SAFETY: Use is restricted to topical in some countries (and not on broken skin). Some consider internal toxicity reports overrated since they may be due to overdose or individual allergic reactions to composite plants. Contains a toxin, helenalin, which can cause gastritis if taken orally in large amounts. Can cause allergic contact dermatitis. Products can be adulterated with Mexican arnica (*Heterotheca inuloides*) and calendula (*Calendula officinalis*). Listed in British and European pharmacopoeias. Granted UK traditional herbal registration by the Medicines and Healthcare Product Regulatory Agency (MHRA).

Capsicum annuum

CAYENNE PEPPER

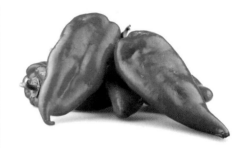

This favorite culinary spice is a prominent pain reliever and its ingredient capsaicin is used in mainstream medicine for topical pain relief.

ABOUT THE PLANT: Native to Mexico, growing in the tropics and subtropics, *Capsicum annuum* is perennial in hot climates and annual in cold. It is a shrub 39 inches (1 m) with small oval leaves, star-like white flowers and distinctive elongated red berries. It prefers warm, nutrient-rich soil and grows and fruits well in pots. Thousands of varieties contain the active ingredient capsaicin.

HISTORY AND FOLKLORE: Brought to Europe in the sixteenth century by Columbus. American medical herbalist John Christopher remarkably said, "In 35 years I have never lost one heart attack patient. . . . if they are still breathing—I pour down them a cup of cayenne tea: a teaspoon of cayenne in a cup of hot water, and within minutes they are up and around." Used in herbal medicine for pain and topically for wounds, bruises, burns, sciatica, neuralgia, and muscle spasms. Also as a stimulant without narcotic effects.

WHAT SCIENTISTS SAY

In humans: In controlled trials cayenne reduces post-shingles neuralgia, HIV, and diabetic neuropathy, and soft tissue and back pain (lumbago). Also reduces headache and joint pain in trials, and plasters reduce postoperative pain requirements and anxiety in children. Also treats tonsillitis, speeds up metabolism, reduces appetite and blood stress markers in obese women, and increased myocardial profusion in a controlled trial.

In the lab: Cayenne's capsaicinoids exhaust a signal linked to pain—a vanilloid receptor (TRPV1) also present in the brain—which itself releases substance P and somatostatin that transmit pain signals to the brain. Capsaicin also depletes substance P, preventing pain signals reaching the brain. Also affects other signals including serotonin, dilates blood vessels, and speeds up metabolism, is anti-inflammatory, antioxidant, and causes the release of endorphins.

KEY INGREDIENTS: The hot pungency of cayenne is due to amines called capsaicinoids such as the active capsaicin (a nonalkaloid nitrogen containing lipid), which together with beta-carotene provides the red color (a chile's potency apparently depends on the length of capsaicin's acid side chain). Also contains oleic, palmitic, and steric acids flavonoids, a volatile oil, and plenty of vitamin C.

HOW TO TAKE IT: For arthritis, medical herbalist Andrew Chevallier recommends 20 drops of cayenne tincture (150 g fresh or 100 g dried plant material in 500 ml 40% alcohol agitated daily for fourteen days, then strained) combined with 100 ml willow bark tincture (same method), 5 ml twice daily. Capsules, plasters, and nasal sprays are also used. Fresh pods, dried pods, and cayenne pepper (not chili powder, which is a mix of cayenne and other spices) can be used in chile oil, the Bloody Mary cocktail, and Mexican-style chocolate ice cream.

SAFETY: Avoid touching the eyes after handling. Do not take seeds on their own. Cayenne can induce stomach irritation, sweating, and runny nose. Not in peptic ulcer, acid indigestion, anal surgery, and skin rashes. Although a foodstuff, some suggest it should not be taken long term, but this may apply to overdosing (regular use can lead to attenuation of burning sensations, and desire for more).

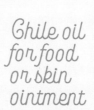

Chile oil for food or skin ointment

It may be simple but it's good.

Chop 3 fresh or dried chiles and stir into ¼ cup (50 ml) olive oil. Add 1 teaspoon ground cayenne pepper if you like it hotter. Keeps in the refrigerator for 3 to 4 days.

Comfrey, chile, and arnica pain-relief ointment

1 cup (250 ml) sunflower oil

10 ounces (300 g) fresh arnica (or 7 ounces (200 g) dried

8 fresh bird's eye chiles, finely chopped

10 ounces (300 g) finely chopped fresh comfrey

3½ ounces (100 g) chopped beeswax

10 drops essential oils of your choice (optional)

The amount and choice of plants can be varied; if you prefer an ointment more targeted at healing skin, use calendula instead of comfrey. This recipe comes from Ross Menzies, long-time medical herbalist at Dilston Physic Garden.

❶ Put the sunflower oil in a nonmetal pan and add the arnica, chiles, and comfrey. Heat very slowly on the lowest heat—do not fry. Ideally, heat gradually for a few hours each day over a couple of days, leaving to cool in between.

❷ Strain through a paper coffee filter, then reheat slowly with the beeswax until melted. Test a little on a teaspoon to see check how firmly it sets. Add extra beeswax as needed to achieve desired solidity on cooling.

❸ Pour into dark jars and allow to cool, with the lids off. If you have used fresh rather than dried plants, when pouring be careful to ensure no water content is added—this will be found as a layer at the bottom of the oil.

❹ When it is partially cooled but not yet solid, you can add 10 drops of an essential oil of your choice such as chamomile or peppermint.

❺ Once the ointment is cool, put the lids on the jars and add a label.

Symphytum officinale

COMFREY

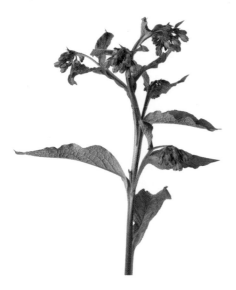

Comfrey is a pretty but coarse-leaved plant that can be a thug in the garden (making it readily available for topical pain relief), with a mass of clinical evidence backing up its centuries-old traditional use.

ABOUT THE PLANT: This European perennial grows to 39 inches (1 m), likes moist habitats, and has large thick, hairy leaves, bell-like white to pink-purple flowers, and a fleshy root. The root is harvested in spring or autumn when its wound-healing chemical allantoin is at its highest.

HISTORY AND FOLKLORE: Long used to heal bruises, sprains, fractures, and broken bones. Sixteenth-century English herbalist Nicholas Culpeper said, "The great comfrey decoction drunk helpeth all inward hurts, bruises, and wounds . . . and for outward wounds and sores in the flesh or sinewy part of the body." It's used by herbalists as a cream for tendon, ligament,

and muscle pain and for fractures, hence its name knitbone. The name comfrey comes from *con firma* meaning the bone is "made firm," and *Symphytum* translates from Greek "to unite." It is grown as a vegetable on the Baltic coast, and the leaf adds a rich flavor to soups and stews, but the root is not recommended internally.

WHAT SCIENTISTS SAY

In humans: Numerous controlled trials and many uncontrolled trials and case studies confirm the traditional use of comfrey species (including *Symphytum officinale* and *S. × uplandicum*) for topical pain relief and for inflammation of muscles and joints. Clinically relieves pain in, for example, sprained ankles (where it is a safe alternative to topical diclofenac), in back pain (where it is an effective aid in combination with the single drug methyl nicotinate), in osteoarthritis, in pressure ulcers, and in abrasion wound healing (including in children over three years old).

A controlled trial compared an ointment made from a root extract of comfrey to diclofenac gel in the treatment of sprained ankles in 164 outpatients. Following application four times a day, assessments of several variables were made—pain reaction to pressure, swelling (the circumference of the joint), judgment of impaired movements, consumption of medication (paracetamol), and pain sensation at rest and at movement. As well as being found as efficacious and tolerable as diclofenac gel (by both physician and patient), some of the variables indicated that comfrey extract may be superior to diclofenac gel.

In the lab: The root and its ingredient allantoin are wound-healing in lab models, stimulatory on cell metabolism promoting healthy cell growth, control inflammation, and induce collagen formation. Contains rosmarinic acid which is a strong anti-inflammatory and antioxidant.

KEY INGREDIENTS: The alkaloid allantoin is active and so is a combination of ingredients including the phenolic acids such as rosmarinic acid. Like butterbur, borage, and coltsfoot, comfrey contains pyrrolizidine alkaloids (such as symphytine and pyrrolizidine) known to be hepatotoxic, carcinogenic, and mutagenic when taken at high doses for prolonged periods internally. Also contains the amino acid asparagine, mucilage, tannins, resin, and a volatile oil.

HOW TO TAKE IT: A sprain massage oil of leaves (500 g fresh chopped plant in 750 ml carrier such as almond oil, heated in a glass bowl over boiling water, covered, and simmered 2 to 3 hours, then strained into dark glass bottle). Ointment made with wax and compresses and poultices of leaves also used.

SAFETY: Topical applications are safe. Internal use is banned in the US and certain European countries based on risk of liver toxicity of root, which contains pyrrolizidine alkaloids that are toxic internally, if taken at a high dose long term. The aerial parts contain minute quantities of these alkaloids, and there's no epidemiological evidence of toxicity in those who eat comfrey leaf. The leaf is used internally as a powerful treatment for gastric and duodenal ulcers. Do not mistake the almost identical leaves of foxglove (*Digitalis*) for comfrey—an error that has caused severe poisoning.

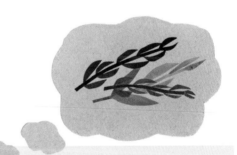

Mindfulness to control pain

This approach for headaches has been used as an alternative therapy for several decades now. It centers on visual imagery of the pain as a distraction.

Focus on the exact location of the pain in your body, what part of the body it is in, and exactly where it is in that area. Estimate its exact size (in cups or plants—is it the size of feverfew, comfrey, or would it fill a willow tree). Now detect what shape it is (in geometric shapes such as a circle or square, or is it a plant—a round flower, a random moss-like shape, a long stalk shape). Then decide what color it is (a deep red, a blue, or white for example). Repeat this sequence over and over.

Many people report that practicing this repeatedly with a headache reduces the intensity of pain, and some that they have been relieved of their headache altogether.

Salix alba

WHITE WILLOW

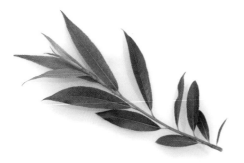

Willow is the source of aspirin (based on the chemical salicin), the most widely used drug in the world. The bark, which is a traditionally used medicine, could make a comeback mainly on account of its superior safety for pain relief.

ABOUT THE PLANT: Native to Europe and western and central Asia, this deciduous tree 30 to 50 feet (9 to 15 m) high thrives in damp regions near water and is one of the most vigorous in rate and type of growth—it sprouts from "whips" (stem cuttings) and even logs. Its gray-brown, deeply fissured bark is used medicinally. Leaves and bark from other willow species (such as *S. fragilis*) are also said to be medicinal.

HISTORY AND FOLKLORE: The bark, used as medicine for joint pain, headaches, gout, lumbago, sciatica, inflammation, and fevers for thousands of years, was first mentioned in Egyptian medical texts from about 1550 BC. Used since then by Greeks and Romans including Hippocrates (who recommended chewing it, drinking leaf tea, or mashing leaves with pepper to drink with wine for relief of fever and pain) and by Pliny and Galen as an

analgesic and antipyretic (reducing fever). This use of willow bark (and of meadowsweet, which contains the same key chemical, salicylic acid) led to salicin being isolated from willow bark in 1838 and synthesized in France in 1853. Aspirin (acetylsalicylic acid) was first made in 1897 by the Bayer Company. To the Taoists the tree represented strength in weakness.

WHAT SCIENTISTS SAY

In humans: The few controlled clinical trials on willow bark (as opposed to aspirin itself) show it reduces lower back pain, joint pain, and treats osteoarthritis. One study suggests willow bark (standardized to 240 mg salicin) is as effective as a synthetic (nonsteroidal anti-inflammatory) drug rofecoxib when given for over six months to 114 people with lower back pain, and is half the cost.

In the lab: Pain-relieving and anti-inflammatory willow bark is associated with multiple actions, prostaglandin regulation, and the lowering of multiple inflammatory mediators (like cytokines and COX2). Shown as good as, if not more effective than, aspirin in lab models of these markers, and a better antioxidant than aspirin on a weight for weight basis of salicin.

KEY INGREDIENTS: Although commercial willow bark extracts are generally standardized to salicin, other ingredients including other salicylates and polyphenols (such as tannins and flavonoids) are responsible for the therapeutic effects.

HOW TO TAKE IT: Fresh or dried bark can be made into a decoction—20 g dried (or 40 g fresh) finely chopped in 750 ml water simmered to 500 ml water, take 120 ml

3 times daily. Bark can also be chewed, and tinctures, capsules, and tablets (which may contain other anti-inflammatory plants) are also used. Willow bark takes longer to act but effects last longer than aspirin. Pollen-laden male catkins infused in vodka (willow schnapps) is a favorite with the Danes.

SAFETY: In contrast to aspirin, willow bark does not irritate the gastrointestinal tract (salicin in willowbark is absorbed in the duodenum rather than the stomach). Caution with anticoagulants in doses above 240 mg salicin/day; at lower doses willow bark does not have the same cardiac and stroke (anticoagulant) preventative actions of aspirin (and an extract dose with 240 mg salicin had no major impact on blood clotting). Caution allergic reactions in salicylate-sensitive individuals and, like aspirin, not for children—although Germany's Commission E states there is no evidence that willowbark preparations should be contraindicated in small children due to the risk of Reye's syndrome, since the salicylates in willowbark are metabolized differently from aspirin. Caution with other anti-inflammatory medicine as additive effects are theoretically possible. Salicylates are not advised in pregnancy.

Tanacetum parthenium

FEVERFEW

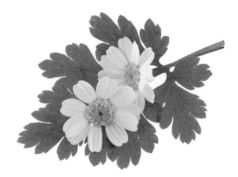

In European herbal medicine feverfew has been used to treat migraine, fever, and arthritis for centuries, and has been shown to be a clinically effective prophylactic medicine for migraine headaches.

ABOUT THE PLANT: With pale green ovate leaves and daisy-like flowers, feverfew grows to 28 inches (70 cm) and looks like overgrown chamomile. This Asian native has now spread across Europe, Australia, and North America, likes the sun and well-drained soil, and blooms all summer. Leaves are harvested when the plant is in flower.

HISTORY AND FOLKLORE: Used historically to reduce fever and all types of pain including rheumatism, and the prevention of migraines. It is said that the wife of a Welsh doctor being cured by a course of feverfew after fifty years of migraines triggered research in the UK in the 1980s, when it became popular for migraines. It was also historically used by physicians in North America as a tonic and for "those who have taken opium too liberally."

WHAT SCIENTISTS SAY

In humans: Several (but not all) controlled clinical trials show feverfew is effective in the prevention of migraine without adverse effects. Later studies with standardization of extracts and dose are more supportive. Feverfew taken with ginger and also in a controlled trial with white willow (*Salix alba*) relieves migraine.

In the lab: Parthenolide, the main terpene ingredient, selectively inhibits an inflammatory agent (NF-kappaB activation) specific to migraines, and affects the signal serotonin, which has been associated with migraine. Extracts are anti-inflammatory in several models of inflammation, and also inhibit prostaglandin synthesis. Flower extract is analgesic, relieving inflammatory and neuropathic pain in lab models.

KEY INGREDIENTS: The sesquiterpene lactone (a signature ingredient of the daisy family) parthenolide is a key active (though feverfew extracts are still potent anti-inflammatories when this chemical is removed because of its skin-sensitizing effects). Certain varieties of feverfew are rich in this constituent, while in others its absence may explain some of the differences in clinical trials. Contains other sesquiterpenes, flavonoids, and a camphorous volatile oil.

HOW TO TAKE IT: Eating 2 to 3 fresh leaves a day to prevent migraine is recommended by British medical herbalist Andrew Chevallier. Tincture and capsules. Poultices for joint aches.

SAFETY: Except in individual allergic reaction (where it can cause mouth ulcers), feverfew is safe and recorded side effects are mild and transient. Parthenolide is a skin sensitizer. No restriction on long-term use. In theory caution in anticoagulants due to inhibition of platelet aggregation, though this has not been shown clinically. Do not take in pregnancy.

Aloe vera syn. *A. barbadensis*

ALOE VERA

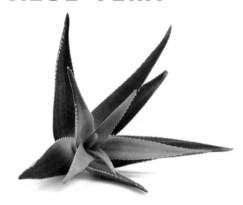

Familiar to many, with its exotic cactus-like leaves, this plant is one of the most widely used anti-inflammatories, especially for skin conditions.

ABOUT THE PLANT: Native to east and southern Africa but growing in the tropics across the world, this perennial is often mistaken for a cactus. It is not frost hardy but thrives as an indoor plant in colder climes. A stemless or short-stemmed succulent with thick, serrated fleshy leaves 2 feet (60 cm)long, gathered into a rosette at the apex with tall yellow or orange flowers, it propagates easily from new buds. *A. saponaria* has also been studied medicinally.

HISTORY AND FOLKLORE: An ancient medicine with records of its use dating back to the Ebers Papyrus (a record of ancient Egyptian medicine in the sixteenth century BC). English herbalist Gerard said about its gastric uses: "When all purging medicines are hurtfull to the stomacke, Aloes onely is comfortable," and about external use, including the eyes "forasmuch as it clenseth and drieth without biting." Near Mecca, aloe is planted beside graves, its name in Arabic meaning patience, referring to the period between death and resurrection. Used in plant medicine today as an anti-inflammatory and pain reliever for arthritis, gingivitis, gout, dermatitis, sunburn, and peptic ulcers.

WHAT SCIENTISTS SAY

In humans: Aloe vera gel is analgesic in tissue damage and postoperative pain in controlled trials, where it is also effective in wound healing, burns, psoriasis, diaper rash, herpes, and wrinkles, and reduces radiation-induced mucositis. Aloe vera is also antidiabetic and hypolipidaemic.

In the lab: It is anti-inflammatory, treats neuropathic and tissue damage pain in lab models, is antioxidant, antimicrobial, and antitumor.

KEY INGREDIENTS: The yellow-brown bitter glycosides known as anthraquinones, aloins A (barbaloin), and B (isobarbaloin) are in its latex, as well as saponins, lectins, terpenes, and alkaloids.

HOW TO TAKE IT: Fresh leaf gel applied topically and added to skin ointments and lotions, shampoo, and shaving creams. For internal use the juice is expressed from the gel and added to food products such as yogurt. The commercial juice has the dark-colored bitter aloins removed. Aloe is a constituent of amaro (meaning bitter), an Italian liqueur.

SAFETY: Considered safe applied topically but not to open wounds or severe burns. Evidence of some gastrointestinal side effects (such as cramps) if taken internally. Carcinogenic effects at high doses in lab models have led to warnings about excessive or long-term internal use. Ensure you have the correct species (there are over 500 species and some aloes can be poisonous). Do not use in pregnancy or breastfeeding.

Making a tussy mussy

Distraction and focus are thought to help ease the perception of pain. Concentrate on picking and preparing a tussy mussy made from pain balms such as arnica, feverfew, comfrey, and willow—and add chile fruits for color. Cut the plants in 4- to 6-inch (10 to 15 cm) lengths. Strip the bottom leaves and rest the plants in a glass of water while you work. Choose a flower for the center in one hand and surround it with a suitable layer of filler plants until you have a tight little bouquet that looks cute and has focused your mind.

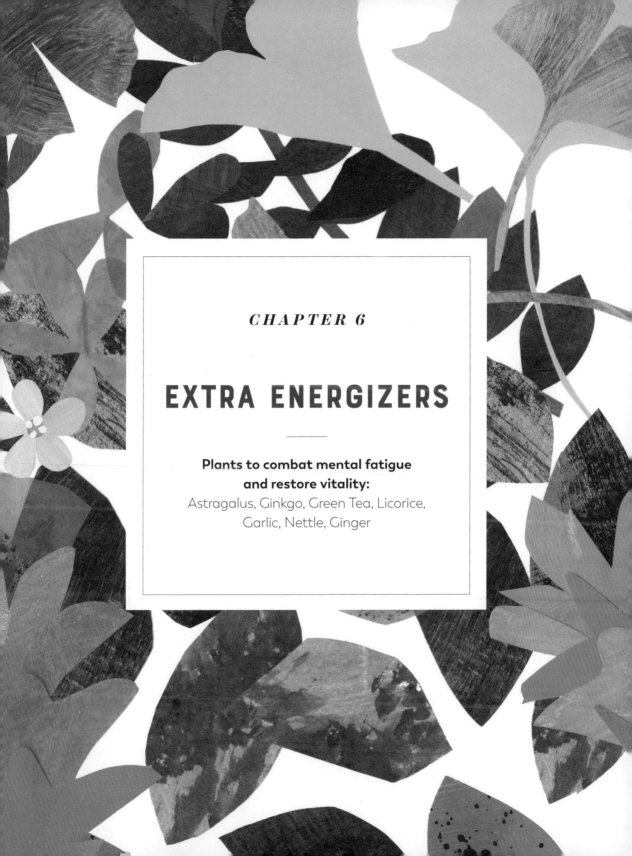

CHAPTER 6

EXTRA ENERGIZERS

**Plants to combat mental fatigue
and restore vitality:**
Astragalus, Ginkgo, Green Tea, Licorice,
Garlic, Nettle, Ginger

Overwhelmed by demands on your time, stretched to the limit, and pounded by sensory overload? For many of us, mental and physical fatigue goes with today's lifestyle and expresses itself through stress, irritability or altered mood and also by physical signs including headaches and gastrointestinal problems. Fortunately, the right plant can boost mental and physical energy by helping to strengthen overstressed body systems.

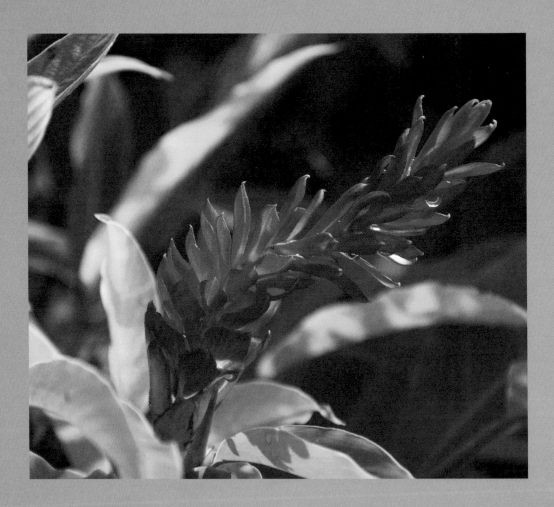

In this chapter we focus on nerve tonics that can combat mental fatigue and increase mental clarity. Our core energizers include two traditional medicinal plants (astragalus and ginkgo), which have origins in China, two European plants, one sweet and the other with a sting (licorice and nettle), a Chinese and Indian spice (ginger), a fiery Asian vegetable (garlic), and a celebrated "superfood" (green tea). We'll also highlight a handful of plants that deliver a range of health benefits by stimulating beneficial actions within the brain. Plants can be energizers that reduce fatigue, tonics that strengthen relevant body systems, or adaptogens that restore stress systems that go out of kilter. Although few plants have been tested in human trials for mental fatigue, lab-based scientific studies show the impact of our energizer balms, or their chemical ingredients, on the brain and nervous system.

Other botanical brain balms that improve energy and mental fatigue are ashwaghanda, an adaptogen that clinically boosts mood, memory, stamina, and much more, and cocoa, which lowers fatigue and relieves symptoms of chronic fatigue syndrome (CFS). Traditionally used energizers that have attracted scientific attention are European oak (*Quercus robur*) and bilberry (*Vaccinium myrtillus*), the Chinese angelica (*Angelica sinensis*), and the famous but endangered snow lotus (*Saussurea involucrata)* from the Himalayas.

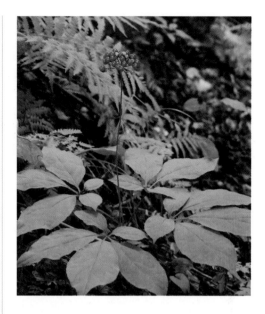

TRADITIONAL CHINESE MEDICINAL PLANTS AND ENERGY

Traditional Chinese medicine (TCM) continues to be practiced on an equal basis alongside orthodox medicines in China today. TCM sees the concept of "vitality" as an essential component of health and healing. Chinese people understand good health as being critically dependent on what they term *qi*, or energy. They describe qi as a natural life force which, if not flowing freely due to an obstruction or block, results in a weaker body.

Ginseng and astragalus are used in traditional Chinese medicine to maintain or restore qi, and traditional ideas on the difference between the two plants are fascinating. Ginseng is said to "nourish vitality" and rescue energy collapse by restoring "yang," and is often used to treat shock. Men in particular recognize it as an energizer and as an aphrodisiac, too. Astragalus, on the other hand, is said to reinforce loss of vitality in what is referred to as "insecurity of the exterior," and is used to help patients counter signs of

Opposite: The root of *Zingiber officinale* (ginger) is valued for a number of medicinal uses including increased vitality.
Above: The root of *Panax ginseng* (ginseng) is used in Chinese medicine to restore *qi* (energy).

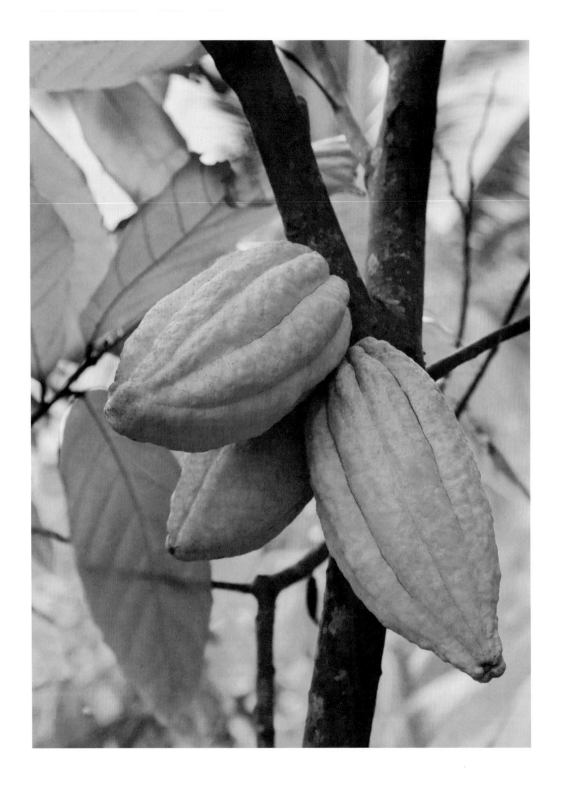

YOUR BRAIN ON PLANTS

weakness and debilitating physical conditions. Sometimes called female ginseng, it is used to help fight stress and disease, too.

Trying to understand how these plants work in terms of conventional Western medicine, especially biological mechanisms, is challenging! Ideas range from the mopping up of tissue-damaging free radicals (antioxidants) and increasing blood flow to countering the adrenal stress response or strengthening brain functions. The energizing plants in our portfolio have many such benefits, and what scientists are prepared to say focuses on brain or nerve cell effects.

We have no research of our own to back up reports on the revitalizing qualities of any of these energizing plants, but love the seasonal plants in our physic garden that act as tonics. Nettle tea or soup, made in spring with added wild garlic, seems to be both energizing and restorative, while combating mental fatigue and sharpening mental clarity, too—but these are our subjective, not scientific, observations.

PLANTS THAT STIMULATE WITH CAFFEINE

With the notable exception of green tea, we have omitted plants which stimulate through their caffeine content. The alkaloid caffeine occurs naturally in some sixty plant species, among which the best known are cocoa beans, kola nuts, tea leaves, and coffee beans. And while caffeine helps people to stay awake and be more alert (it blocks the sleep-inducing brain

Opposite: *Theobroma cacao* (cocoa) stimulates through its caffeine content and relieves fatigue but can produce unwelcome symptoms, too.
Below: We've observed tea of *Urtica urens* (nettle) to be a restorative tonic when taken at Dilston Physic Garden.

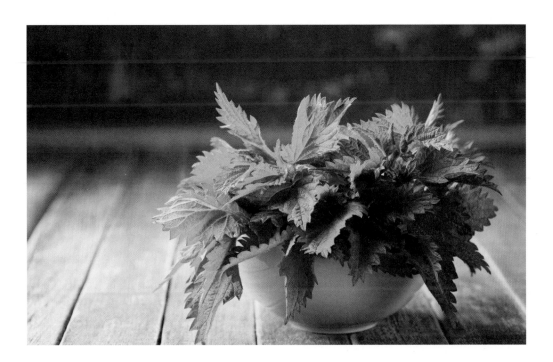

signal adenosine), it is not ideal for everyone, especially if used in large amounts. In some people caffeine provokes unwelcome nervous symptoms such as insomnia and/or migraine as well as cardiac effects including irregular heart rhythms.

TRADITIONAL ENERGIZER BALMS BACKED BY EXPLORATORY SCIENCE

Plants reputed to maintain mental or physical stamina include betel nut (*Areca catechu*) chewed in India as a digestive, damiana (*Turnera diffusa*), gotu kola (*Centella asiatica*), Indian mulberry (*Morinda citrifolia*), an orchid (*Dendrobium officinale*), magnolia vine (*Schisandra propinqua* subsp. *sinensis*), sarsaparilla (*Smilax sarsaparilla*), and the European slippery elm bark (*Ulmus rubra*). We highlight two plants used in traditional Chinese medicine and two used by Western medical herbalists as being of particular interest.

Chinese angelica (*Angelica sinensis*) has long been used in traditional Chinese medicine for increasing energy. It has been shown in lab models to improve exercise performance and protect against physical fatigue. Known as female ginseng (as is astragalus) it may have estrogenic effects and is best not used by men.

Snow lotus (*Saussurea involucrata, S. laniceps,* and other species) is a traditional energizer. Lab tests show that the beautiful and endangered white-flowered snow lotus

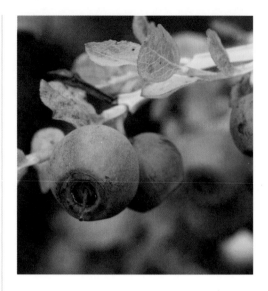

reduces fatigue and stress effects (among many other health benefits recorded in Tibetan and Chinese medicine). Extracts extend stamina in lab models as well as having antioxidant, immunomodulatory, antiaging, and neuroprotective actions.

Bilberry (*Vaccinium myrtillus*) is closely related to the blueberry (*Vaccinium corymbosum*). The European native bilberry is used by Western medical herbalists for people with CFS, and its flavonoid anthocyanin chemicals have neuroprotective effects in lab models. Bilberry and its main constituents also have neuroprotective effects against retinal neuronal damage in the lab.

Oak (*Quercus robur*) is sacred to the druids and was venerated by the ancient Greeks. The oak tree is a Celtic symbol of strength, renowned for building long-lasting ships, houses, and furniture. The bark is used by medical herbalists as a tonic, and in one clinical trial relieved symptoms of CFS.

Above: *Vaccinum myrtillus* (bilberry) and *Quercus robur* (oak)
opposite are used by medical herbalists for people with chronic fatigue syndrome.

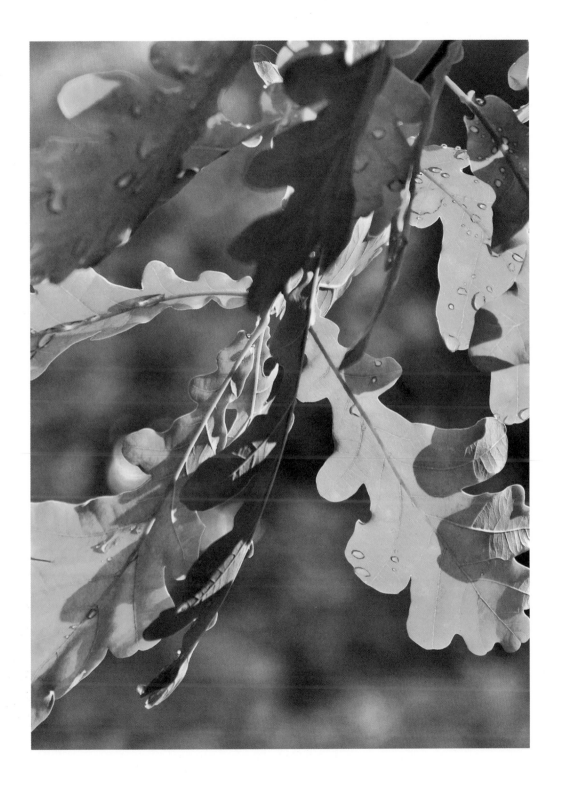

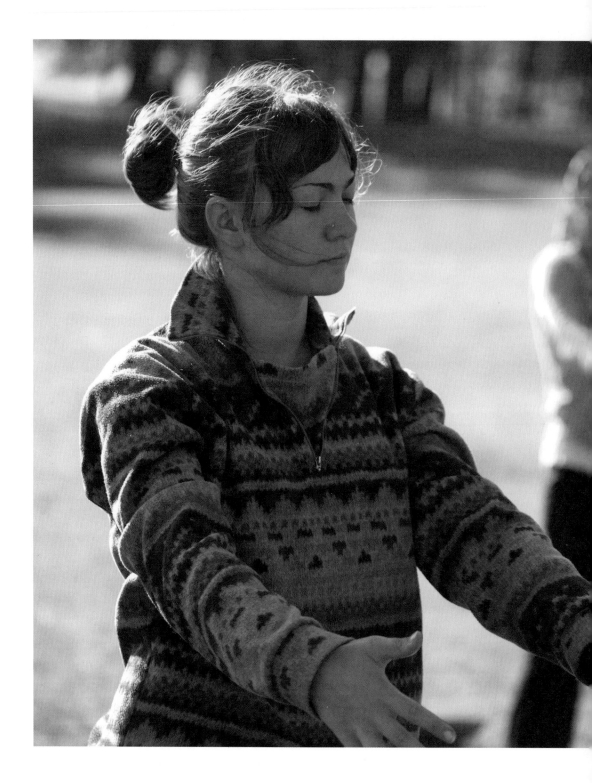

YOUR BRAIN ON PLANTS

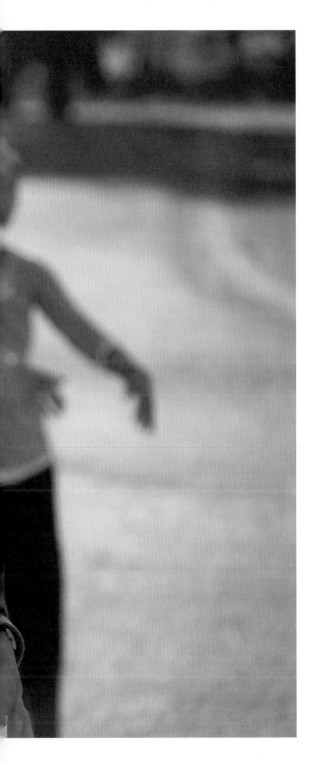

Qi gong with aromatics

Qi gong is the ancient Chinese practice of movement and meditation often performed in groups and designed to enhance health and well-being by controlling the "flow of energy." The gentle exercises are repeated a number of times, usually in a set sequence. They are slow, graceful and involve carefully balanced movements of the whole body.

Health benefits in initial controlled trials include relieving migraine headaches and other pain, improving the immune system, and reducing stress and depression. Most intriguing perhaps are growth effects on cells in culture (lymphocyte immune cells), which have been recorded to grow in test situations under the influence of a qi gong master.

One cross-population study and several controlled trials assessing overall health status showed that qi gong improves various scores including physical function, quality of life, immune function, and psychological symptoms compared to sedentary individuals and to those taking other forms of exercise. This suggests we have much still to learn about the physical basis of energy and bodily health.

Once you have learned the movements from a qualified teacher who has been trained by a qi gong master, try practicing near a bed of an energizing aromatic plants or dab a few drops of essential oil from them on your collar. You will feel your mental and physical vitality increase.

Astragalus mongholicus syn. *A. membranaceus*

ASTRAGALUS

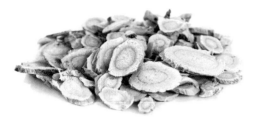

This Chinese medicinal plant of ancient origin is an important tonic used to restore *qi* (vital energy). It improves energy, and studies support its use as an immune booster and cortisol (stress hormone) controller in traditional Chinese medicine, and a tonic and immunostimulant in Western herbal medicine.

ABOUT THE PLANT: Native to Korea, China and Mongolia, *Astragalus mongholicus* is the main astragalus species used medically. It is a perennial plant growing to 16 inches (10 cm) with yellow flowers and a root (the part used for medicinal purposes) covered with a yellowish wrinkled skin.

HISTORY AND FOLKLORE: Known as huang-qi and used in China for 2,000 years, it was first recorded in *Shen Nong Ben Cao Jing* (*The Divine Farmer's Materia Medica*) where it was regarded as a remedy for fatigue and lack of vitality, especially in young people. Li Shizhen, a famous scholar in the Ming dynasty regarded as the father of Chinese medicine, extolled its virtues as the "leader of all tonics." In the West it was also known as milk vetch, and the sixteenth-century British physician and herbalist William Turner referred to it as "milk lentil," because "it hath leaves like lentils and the power to make much milk."

WHAT SCIENTISTS SAY

In humans: Initial controlled clinical trials conducted in China show astragalus helps chronic fatigue and cancer sufferers recover from fatigue, and also helps stroke sufferers, where it improves cognitive function. In a pilot trial it raises IQ in young people with ADHD (comparable to Ritalin) when combined with other traditional Chinese medicine plants. It is also an immunostimulant and increases antioxidant markers in controlled trials.

In the lab: Astragalus is neuroprotective, prevents nerve cell damage after exposure to toxic levels of the stimulatory signal (glutamate), and promotes nerve cell regeneration. It lowers anxiety, is anticonvulsant, protects against brain injury (such as in ischemia or edema), and improves memory in different models. As well as being anti-inflammatory, antioxidant, and immunostimulant, its flavonoids relieve chronic fatigue syndrome in lab models.

KEY INGREDIENTS: Saponins such as astragalosides and flavonoids, phytosterols (such as sitosterol), amino and fatty acids and an essential oil.

HOW TO TAKE IT: The dried root is commonly made into a decoction (20 g per 750 ml water, simmered to 500 ml, daily) and often mixed with black tea. Root is licorice-like and is used in cooking in China, the sliced root being added to soups (chicken or fish) with other herbs added for flavor. Also taken in liquid extract, tincture, powder, capsules, or tablets.

SAFETY: Widely regarded as safe but theoretically not recommended with drugs that suppress the immune system. Contraindicated in acute infection. Not enough information for use in pregnancy and breastfeeding. Astragalus is in the Chinese and Japanese pharmacopoeias and is available as a dietary supplement in the USA and Australia.

Ginkgo biloba

GINKGO

Gingko is sometimes referred to as a living

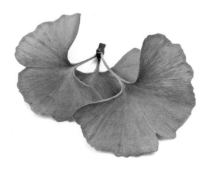

fossil; its present form is practically unchanged from fossils of gingko found in rocks from the Jurassic and Cretaceous periods. Originally used medicinally by the Chinese, its ability to counter fatigue, including mental "fog," is attributed to it reducing oxidative stress and promoting blood flow.

ABOUT THE PLANT: This deciduous tree from central China grows up to 98 feet (30 m). It can live for thousands of years and will survive (but not bear fruit) in colder climates. Ginkgo's distinctive fan-shaped green to yellow leaves are bi-lobed (hence *biloba*) and the nuts that form inside the unpleasant-smelling flesh of its fruit are considered delicious, nutritious, and the most medicinal part of the plant.

HISTORY AND FOLKLORE: To the ancient Chinese, ginkgo was primarily a symbol of longevity and vitality (and, with its male and female trees, a manifestation of their philosophy of yin and yang). Many Taoist temple courtyards feature gingko trees that are thousands of years old. In Japan, ginkgo trees were the only plants to survive the Hiroshima atomic bomb and are still alive there today. It was first used medicinally in China in the tenth century and in Germany in the 1960s. Ginkgo is now widely cultivated and provides a best-selling plant medicine in France and Germany.

WHAT SCIENTISTS SAY

In humans: Initial controlled clinical trials indicate that leaf extracts improve endurance performance (aerobic exercise) and relieve both fatigue and depression in the elderly. Although evidence is controversial, extracts generally improve cognitive function (where they may be more effective at higher doses) and quality of life in controlled trials in people with CFS, MS, and dementia. In one review of four dietary supplements (including ginseng) for mental energy, the evidence favored ginkgo for improvements in attention and mood.

In the lab: Protects from inflammatory and oxidative stress (such as preventing free radical damage) and blood clotting (it inhibits platelet activating factor, which helps blood clot). Also neuroprotective in several models, and increases blood flow and tissue oxygenation (vasoactive) and the feel-good and memory brain signals dopamine, serotonin (inhibits monoamine oxidase), and acetylcholine. Also interacts with calming (GABA) receptors.

KEY INGREDIENTS: The terpene trilactones ginkgolides (A, B, C, and J) and bilobalide, as well as flavonoid glycosides (and their products such apigenin) and proanthocynanidins.

HOW TO TAKE IT: Commonly taken as tablets or tinctures. May need to be taken for six months to have effects. Fresh or dried leaves are also taken as teas. Nuts are used (up to a maximum of five a day) in cooking and they are regarded as a delicacy by the Chinese.

SAFETY: Nuts should not be consumed over five a day. Pungent flesh coating around seeds may cause sensitivity. Leaves contain an inhibitor of a factor (platelet activating factor) involved in coagulation, and among contraindications are with anticoagulants (though controlled studies do not confirm this), antidepressants, and anticonvulsants. Side effects include nausea, restlessness, and increased risk of bleeding, and therefore potentially contraindicated in surgery (though studies show it does not affect clotting times). Not enough evidence for use in pregnancy.

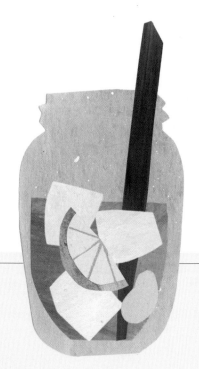

Moscow mule

The energy-boosting, plant-infused cocktail

Ice cubes
½ lime
1½ ounces (40 ml) vodka (with several slices of peeled fresh ginger and astragalus root, and chopped licorice sticks steeped in it for 1 or 2 weeks, agitating daily)
1 teaspoon agave syrup, if required
1 bottle ginger beer
1 stick licorice root to stir

Fill a large round or tall glass with ice, squeeze the lime over it, and pop the lime in the glass. Add the flavored vodka (and syrup to taste) and fill with ginger beer. Add a slice of fresh ginger and a stick of licorice to stir.

Camellia sinensis syn. *Thea sinensis*

GREEN TEA

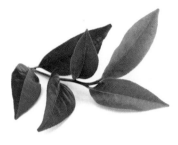

Among the many health benefits of green tea, leaves improve mental strength and function and offset the mental and physical fatigue associated with today's stressful lifestyles.

ABOUT THE PLANT: An evergreen shrub or small tree with shiny leaves and yellow white flowers, *C. sinensis* originates from China. Green tea comes from the same plant as black and oolong teas—the difference is that its leaves are not darkened by oxidization. Cultivated in tropical or subtropical climates, the bush also survives in temperate zones, and tea is now produced in the UK.

HISTORY AND FOLKLORE: Leaves were chewed more than 3,000 years ago in China to sustain vitality. The first historic mention of tea, referred to as *cha* in Lu Yu's *The Classics of Tea*, dates back to 2737 BC, when Emperor Shennong (a beacon of wisdom and medical knowledge) was said to have drunk hot water into which *Camellia* leaves had accidentally fallen and found it so refreshing he requested it from then on. Green tea was the first type of tea drunk and it is still at the center of the Japanese tea ceremony, which uses infused matcha, or *matsu-cha* (powdered green tea).

WHAT SCIENTISTS SAY

In humans: Green tea extract (containing epigallocatechin-3-gallate or EGCG) enhanced cognitive learning in young people with Down's syndrome, and also attention and relaxation in normal adults. In controlled trials the amino acid found in green tea, l-theanine, lowered anxiety and raised blood pressure in stress-prone adults, and in a pilot trial showed benefits on anxiety, sleep, and cognitive impairment in major depression. Green tea, and l-theanine, improve memory and attention in mild cognitive impairment, and green tea also improves cognitive function and reduces blood oxidative stress markers in Alzheimer's. In cross-section population (epidemiological) studies in Japan, psychological stress is lower in people who drink it compared to those who do not.

In the lab: Extracts high in catechins (flavonoids) relieve fatigue in models of CFS (supporting the idea that it offsets mental fatigue due to catechins and not the stimulant caffeine), relieve cognitive dysfunction, and catechins affect cannabinoid signals. It also has key antioxidant and anti-inflammatory actions.

KEY INGREDIENTS: Polyphenols, predominantly flavonoids such as catechin and EGCG—the most abundant and considered most bioactive ingredient, along with the amino acid l-theanine. Also contains caffeine (1 to 5%), theobromine and theophylline (the xanthene alkaloids also in chocolate), tannins, and vitamin C.

HOW TO TAKE IT: Favored as a tea for thousands of years, and little else compares (8 to 10 cups daily suggested for a medicinal dose), though it is used in marinades, glazes, ice cream, and sweets. Leaves from the pink-blossomed *C. sasanqua* species make a perfectly palatable tea that tastes like Japanese green tea. Using a lower temperature of water (140 to 194°F/ 60 to 90°C) creates a higher taste quality, and in Japan, tea is often drunk from repeat infusions of the same leaves. Also taken as capsules and as a powder.

SAFETY: Moderate consumption is safe, even during pregnancy, but excessive use may adversely affect the gut and liver and, due to tannin content, may affect concurrent iron absorption. With around 100 mg caffeine per cup, decaffeinated is recommended for the caffeine sensitive and in hypertension, cardiac arrhythmias, anxiety disorders, and insomnia. Excessive consumption may interact with anticoagulants.

Glycyrrhyza glabra syn. *Liquiritia officinalis*

LICORICE

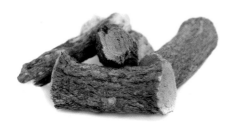

The ingredient of one of the world's favorite sweets, licorice is used for fatigue, particularly adrenal stress, and has protective effects on brain cells. It is often used to disguise the bitter tastes of Western plant medicines or drugs with sweetness.

ABOUT THE PLANT: A perennial from Eurasia, northern Africa, and western Asia, it likes full sun and does not survive winter in colder regions. Growing to 5 feet (1.5 m) with pinnate leaves and pale pink-purple flowers, it is the roots (stolons or suckers) that are harvested and dried in autumn for use as sticks.

HISTORY AND FOLKLORE: The botanical name comes from the Greek for sweet and root, and around 2000 BC the Egyptian pharaohs chewed sticks and took it as a sweet drink. It was used in the first century by physician Dioscorides, who told Roman soldiers to chew the root to allay thirst. Also known as *gan cao* in traditional Chinese medicine, it is believed to harmonize other ingredients in a formula. Used in traditional Japanese medicine and in Ayurvedic medicine for rejuvenation, and by Western medical herbalists for adrenal insufficiency and as a restorative tonic (being immunostimulant, anti-inflammatory, antiviral and antibacterial). Researched since the 1950s for its major clinical efficacy in gastric and duodenal ulceration.

WHAT SCIENTISTS SAY

In humans: As part of a traditional Chinese medicine formula (*baoyuan dahuang*), extracts relieve fatigue in patients with kidney disease, and in controlled trials it is more effective than HRT in reducing hot flushes in menopausal women. Was successful in a case study for CFS.

In the lab: Inhibits fatigue and enhances memory in lab models as well as protecting against oxidative stress and inflammation, and is neuroprotective in cultured cells and in models of brain injury (such as restricted blood flow). Reduces oxidative stress in the hippocampus (a key memory area in the brain) and is also active as an antidepressant and in generating new nerve cells (neurogenesis).

KEY INGREDIENTS: The triterpene glycosides (saponins) such as glycyrrhizin acid, which accounts for sweet flavor (said to be 50 times sweeter than sugar). Also contains flavonoids (such as liquiritin), responsible for the root's yellow color, as well as sterols, coumarins and an essential oil.

HOW TO TAKE IT: Decoction of peeled or unpeeled root (20 g per 750 ml water, simmered to 500 ml) is commonly taken daily. Fresh root also made into a paste or dried juice stick. Dried root can be chewed, and fresh or dried root made into a tincture or liqueur. Also taken as capsules. As an ingredient in confectionery, its sweetness is less harsh and longer-lasting than sugar and it doesn't damage teeth (licorice lollipops actually protect children's teeth) or raise blood glucose.

SAFETY: Considered safe within upper dose limit of 600 mg active ingredient glycyorrhizin per day. Contraindicated in heart disease, high blood pressure, fluid retention, with oral and topical corticosteroids and, in theory, with anticoagulants and with oral contraceptives in a high dose or with long-term use (glycyrrhetic acid can accumulate). An awareness of steroid effects (elevated blood cortisol) is advised. Caution in pregnancy.

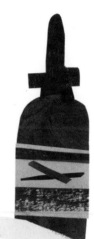

Bellows breath (Bhastrika)

A number of studies investigated the beneficial effects of breathing techniques on physiological and mental conditions including fatigue. This yogic technique is said to increase energy.

Place 10 drops of licorice or ginger essential oil on a saucer and rest it on your lap. Sit up comfortably and elongate and align the spine and head, bringing your chin back.

Breathe deeply and forcefully through your nose (both nostrils) inhaling and exhaling equally (about a second each) to establish a rhythm. Repeat this ten times, then inhale completely and hold your breath for one to five seconds, before exhaling completely. You can do five rounds or more as you wish, with a break in between.

Nettle and wild garlic soup

Serves 3 to 4

Knob of butter or dollop of olive oil or
   coconut oil

1 onion, finely chopped

1 carrot, finely chopped

1 celery stick, finely chopped

2 to 3 small potatoes, sliced

1 teaspoon chopped fresh ginger
   (optional)

1 to 2 teaspoons ground turmeric or
   chopped fresh turmeric

1 quart (1 L) vegetable stock

14 ounces (400 g) nettle tips and
   garlic leaves, chopped

Salt and pepper to taste

This is a lovely tonic and Dilston favorite that we serve up to garden volunteers who come to prepare the physic garden for its influx of spring visitors. Both nettles and wild garlic send up new leaves in early spring. Pick the youngest garlic leaves and (wearing gloves) the tips of nettles before they are more than about 12 inches (30 cm) high.

❶ Heat the butter, olive oil, or coconut oil in a large saucepan over a medium heat. Add the onion, carrot, celery, potatoes, and ginger if using, and cook for 10 minutes.

❷ Add the turmeric and vegetable stock and cook for 10 to 15 minutes more until the potatoes are soft.

❸ Add the nettle and garlic leaves to the pan and cook for 5 minutes more.

❹ Remove from the heat, puree in a blender, and add salt and freshly ground pepper to taste.

❺ Serve with either cream, grated parmesan cheese, or a sprinkling of garlic flowers and leaves.

Allium sativum

GARLIC

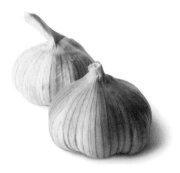

A medicinal plant and food with many health benefits, including antibiotic and cholesterol control, which has more scientific backing for its antifatigue effects than most botanic energizers, and is revered as an antiaging remedy.

ABOUT THE PLANT: This 12 to 39-inch (30 cm to 1 m) herbaceous perennial originates from central Asia. With linear leaves and white or reddish flowers and its distinctive bulb, it is related to wild garlic (*A. ursinum*), which covers north European woodland floors in spring.

HISTORY AND FOLKLORE: Renowned as protection against demons (possibly related to "foul breath" or antibiotic actions), its reputation as an aphrodisiac led to monks of various orders avoiding garlic. It is recorded for its medicinal use over 7,000 years: the second-century Greek physician Galen described it as a cure-all, Gerard was skeptical, and a Mohammedan legend tells of garlic springing up after the devil escaped from the garden of Eden. Using garlic as a tonic was well known in ancient times, and the Egyptians gave it to slaves building the Pyramids, who rebelled when there was a shortage because garlic helped them resist disease, restore energy, and reduce fatigue. In plant medicine today it treats fatigue, and there are claims it increases not only vitality but also longevity.

WHAT SCIENTISTS SAY

In humans: As well as antioxidant, antibiotic, lowering of blood pressure and cholesterol—and cardioprotective effects confirmed in many clinical trials—garlic relieves symptoms in people with physical fatigue, due to a cold or flu for example, suggesting it resolves fatigue in a variety of ways. In Japanese studies on 1,000 human patients with fatigue, depression, and anxiety, garlic extract (with vitamins) reduced all these symptoms in the majority. In patients with stress-related symptoms the same combination relieved general fatigue, headache, dizziness, and appetite loss, among other symptoms.

In the lab: Extracts affect adrenal gland molecules (receptors for the angiotensin hormone) that govern the stress responses and blood pressure. In other models garlic promotes exercise endurance. It is antibiotic, antioxidant and neuroprotective, and extracts and the chemical allicin improve memory.

KEY INGREDIENTS: Vitamins, minerals (high in selenium), sulphur-containing compounds, a volatile oil (with unstable constituents such as alliin that is transformed to allicin on cutting or bruising), as well as amino acids (such as tryptophan and arginine), saponins, and flavonoids.

HOW TO TAKE IT: For health benefits 1 to 3 cloves (10 to 30 g minus skin and roots) best used raw and crushed, or smoked or pickled (which also mellows the flavor). Added to dishes of all kinds from sauces to stews where dose can reach the medicinal level. Fresh leaves, flowers, and seeds of wild garlic (subject of less research but still showing benefits similar to *A. sativum*) are a delicious addition to salads, pesto, and soups. The method of processing garlic is said to affect intensity of antifatigue effect, the most favorable form being bulbs aged for several weeks in a water-ethanol mixture. Capsules and tablets also used.

SAFETY: Well tolerated, with few side effects reported in numerous clinical trials. Caution if taking anticoagulant, antiplatelet, anti-hypertensive and antihyperlipidaemic agents.

Urtica urens

NETTLE

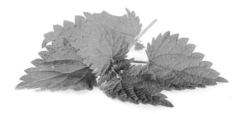

The taste and tonic action of fresh spring nettle tea and soup should overcome reluctance to use this weed with a sting as a medicinal plant. Its use since ancient times as a tonic comes with a series of lab studies showing how it stimulates mood and memory and works as a neuroregenerative.

ABOUT THE PLANT: Originating from Russia, Scandinavia, Europe, and northern Africa, nettle grows to 39 inches (1 m), much to the annoyance of most gardeners. This annual has heart-shaped leaves and green flowers (which are incomplete, with stamens on male and pistils on female flowers). The larger nettle *U. dioica* has similar health uses.

HISTORY AND FOLKLORE: The Latin name *uro* translates as "I burn." Roman soldiers allegedly brought a nettle (*U. pilulifera*) to Britain to chafe their limbs in the cold, the sting stimulating blood supply. Recommended for several ailments by Dioscorides according to J. H. Clarke who writes in *A Dictionary of Practical Materia Medica*, "Being eaten, as Dioscorides saith, boiled with periwinkles, it maketh the body soluble, doing it by a kind of cleansing faculty." The Greek philosopher Platonicus (c. 400 AD) said it would "treat symptoms of feeling cold after being burnt" (burnt is now thought to mean being shocked), and nettle is one of the nine plants used in the Anglo-Saxon "Nine Herb Charm" to counter "poisons" (infection). Recognized today as a stimulating tonic, it is claimed to be a restorative for stressed adrenals. Some medical herbalists say it is particularly useful for those suffering from severe "burnout" that results from profound fatigue, brain fog, chronic pain, and feelings of depression and intense anxiety. Young shoots are cooked and taste like spinach.

WHAT SCIENTISTS SAY

In humans: Clinical trials have not yet focused on mental states but have confirmed other traditional uses such as reducing blood lipids, joint pain, infections, and oxidative stress in diabetics.

In the lab: Nettle reduces oxidative stress in exercise-stressed models and depressive behavior, as well as enhancing cognitive function. Acts on the brain's memory signal (acetylcholine receptors), and in models of encephalopathy (brain disease) nettle increases the number of nerve cells in the memory area of the brain (hippocampus) and also the number of cells (glia) that support nerve cells in the brain. Also antibiotic, anti-inflammatory, and neuroprotective in cell models.

KEY INGREDIENTS: Flavonol glycosides (such as rutin), carotenoids, and histamine, serotonin, and acetylcholine, as well as formic acid in stinging hairs and the coumarin scopolecin in root. High in vitamins C and K, calcium, potassium, and other minerals.

HOW TO TAKE IT: For internal use, pick leaves before flowering to make tea (5 to 12 g fresh or 2 to 6 g dried per 240 ml water). Fresh leaves also used to make pressed juice, salads (in early spring before sting develops), soup, pesto, pasta, and puddings as well as beer, wine, and liqueur. Tinctures, capsules, and dried root also used. Can be used in skin and hair creams (externally) for pain such as arthritic, where the stinging is part of the treatment.

SAFETY: Apart from the hazard of being stung, or if you're allergic to nettle stings, nettle is regarded as free of contraindications, though it is advised to abstain if breastfeeding. Listed in the US pharmacopoeia and freely available as a dietary supplement.

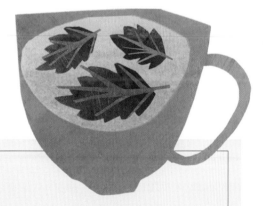

Fresh nettle tea

Gather nettles in the spring before they have flowered. Wear gloves and with scissors cut healthy, leafy stems from the top third of the plant—it's only the leaves you'll use in the tea. Aim to collect about 30 g leaves per 500 ml of water. Once you get home, put the leaves in a colander and rinse them under a cold tap to clear out insects and debris. Then put them in a teapot and pour over freshly boiled water. Allow the leaves to steep until the tea is the strength you prefer, strain into your favorite cup, and prepare to feel revitalized.

Zingiber officinale

GINGER

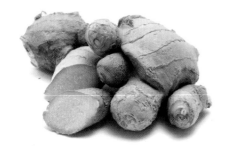

The "spice of life" in Chinese medicine, this root is valued for numerous medicinal uses, for increasing vitality, and particularly as a digestive (as well as for its culinary uses and as an ornamental plant).

ABOUT THE PLANT: From India and south and central China, this perennial grows throughout the tropics to 2 feet (60 cm), with erect lance-shaped leaves, striking spikes of pink buds and yellow flowers, and a yellowish aromatic root (rhizome) harvested in autumn. Needs temperatures above 68°F (20°C) and moist conditions, and can be pot-grown. Other species tested medicinally include *Z. montanum* syn. *Z. purpureum*. Turmeric and hardy ornamental gingers belong to the same plant family, the Zingiberaceae.

HISTORY AND FOLKLORE: Used for thousands of years across many cultures, the root is so widely eaten in India that it is considered a universal medicine. Ayurvedic tradition states that everyone should eat fresh ginger just before lunch and dinner to enhance digestion. In traditional Chinese medicine (which uses the fresh and dried root differently) ginger restores "devastated yang"

associated with fatigue, lack of energy, and cold. Aphrodisiac qualities are mentioned in many cultures, and in Italy's famed University of Salerno medical school it was prescribed for a happy life in old age: "Eat ginger, and you will love and be loved as in your youth." In herbal medicine today it's used for CFS or fatigue in general, to relieve muscle tension, stimulate circulation, enhance memory and attention, and increase appetite and even sexual desire.

WHAT SCIENTISTS SAY

In humans: Apart from many clinical trials that confirm antinausea, antiemetic, and other bodily effects, including topical analgesic, human trials on its mental benefits are in their infancy, but there is one that shows ginger enhanced memory in 60 middle-aged women against a placebo.

In the lab: Among wide-ranging effects on cells and lab models, those relevant to mental fatigue are antioxidant, anti-inflammatory, neuroprotective as well as antibiotic. *Zingiber officinale* (and *Z. purpureum*) prevents oxidative damage to brain cells, including those lost in Alzheimer's (such as hippocampal neurons), improves learning, and reverses memory deficits in aging models associated with nerve growth factor for normal brain development and maintenance. In combination with ginkgo (*Ginkgo biloba*) it lowers anxiety similar to diazepam, and a phenolic compound (dehydrozingerone) is antidepressant via the mood-boosting brain signal (serotonin).

KEY INGREDIENTS: A resin (known as oleoresin) contains two pungent, hot components: sesquiterpenes such as zingiberene and phenolics such as gingerols, which decompose to shogaols on drying. Also contains curcumene, beta-bisabolene, and an essential oil (containing geranial and cineole).

HOW TO TAKE IT: The rhizome (up to 3 g) eaten as raw slices (adding salt and vinegar if necessary) or to make tea (commonly with lemon and turmeric), liqueurs, wine, beer, cordials, and in smoothies, pickles, confectionery and numerous savory and sweet dishes. Also taken as a tincture and capsules. Ginger is a common additive to other medicines.

SAFETY: Generally regarded as safe though can cause heartburn and bloating. Theoretical cautions include anticoagulants, gallstones, gastric ulcers, or reflux. It is in the Chinese, Japanese, Indian, American, European, and British pharmacopoeias and widely available as a dietary supplement.

Right nostril breath (Bedhi)

Yogic breathing is renowned for increasing energy, which makes sense since breathing effectively oxygenates the blood. Try this exercise when you are feeling tired.

Place ten drops of ginger essential oil on a tissue and place on your lap or tuck into your collar. Sit with a straight back, crosslegged or on a chair, and elongate your spine, bringing your chin back to align spine and head.

Take five deep slow breaths though the nose, then close the left nostril and breathe (inhale and exhale) slowly and deeply through the right nostril only. Repeat this ten times. Inhale completely, hold your breath in for one to five seconds, and then exhale completely. You can build this exercise up to 15 minutes of this breathing.

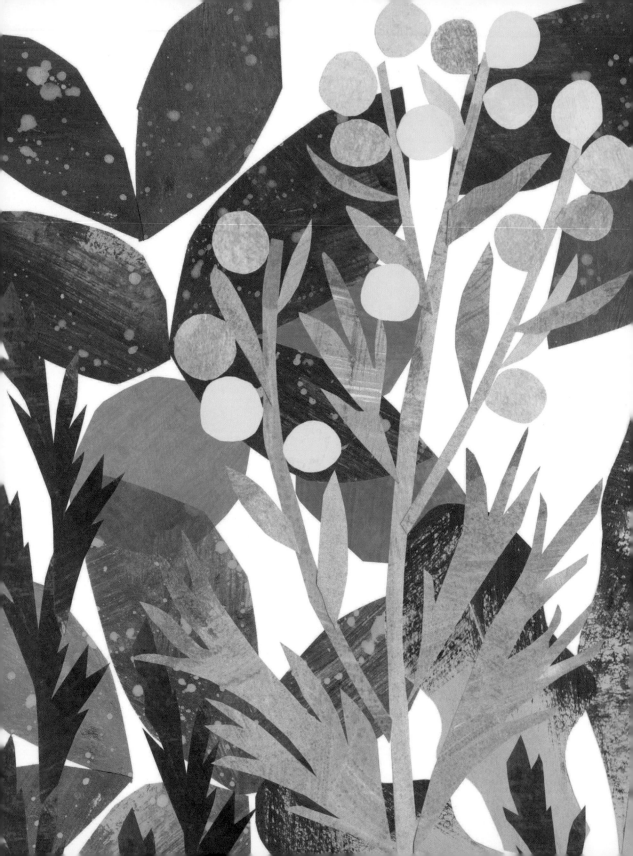

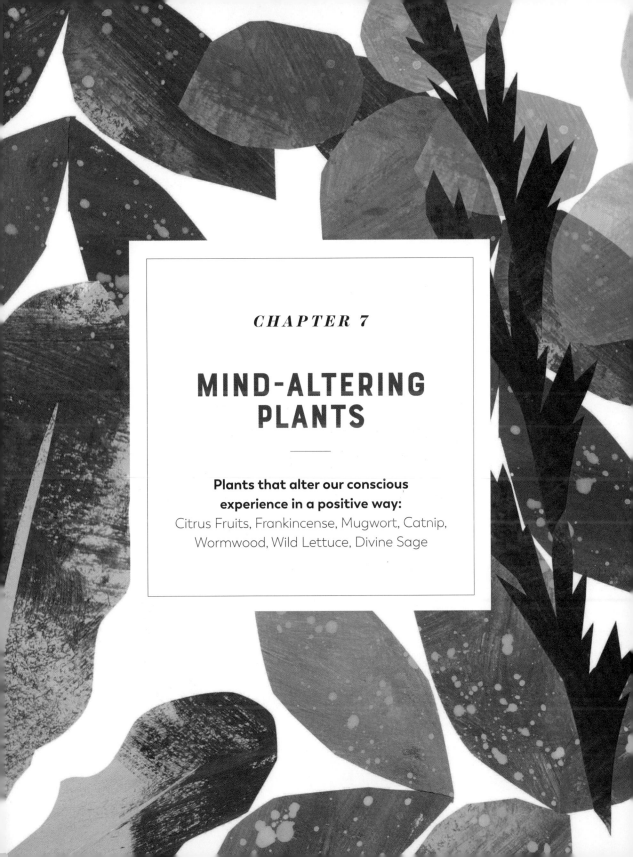

CHAPTER 7

MIND-ALTERING PLANTS

Plants that alter our conscious experience in a positive way:
Citrus Fruits, Frankincense, Mugwort, Catnip, Wormwood, Wild Lettuce, Divine Sage

Exhilaration and inspiration are on many people's wish list, and a number of mind-altering plants can safely (and legally) induce this state. Some say mind-altering plants led to the evolution of a more creative human consciousness and that creativity is closely linked to our survival. There is little research on the consciousness-altering effects but there is research on the effects of these plants on the brain, and this provides clues about how they work to enrich our experience.

At Dilston Physic Garden we divide mind-altering plants into three categories: highly potent, dangerous plants that are never to be used; safer but still potent plants best taken under supervision; and plants with gentler ways of uplifting mood and mind that are safe if you heed the information provided.

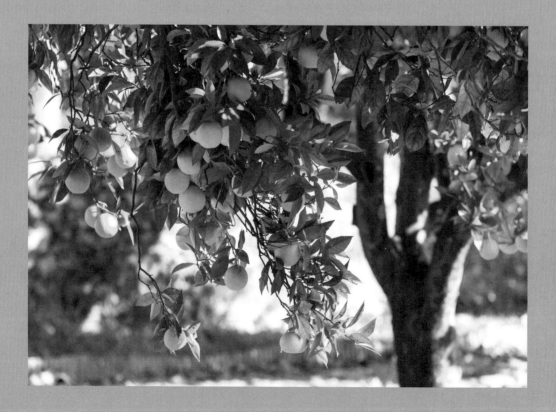

HOW WE GOT HOOKED ON UPLIFT BALMS

During the 1990s our Newcastle University research took an unexpected turn—patients experiencing visual hallucinations of people and animals, known as Lewy body dementia. We looked for clues as to what could be going on in the brain to induce these visions. The answer was found in plants used in rituals to induce visions, for example mandrake and belladonna, which contain a chemical that blocks the brain signal acetylcholine, connected with memory. In the dementia patients it became clear that loss of this signal was linked to their visions. So we learned more about the treatment of people with the condition and about consciousness itself, and were helped in our understanding by plants. Fascinated by all the folklore surrounding such psychedelic but often toxic plant species (belladonna is not called deadly nightshade for nothing), we obtained other mind-altering, though much safer, plants and cultivated them at Dilston Physic Garden.

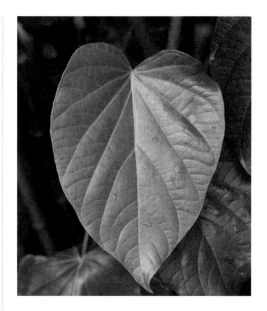

THE MIND-ALTERING BRAIN SIGNALS

The majority of plants that alter our conscious experience affect pleasure (serotonin, dopamine, and noradrenaline), pain and perception (opioid and cannabinoid), and calming (GABA) signals, but they can also affect attention (acetylcholine) signals. It's highly likely that other effects on brain signals are still to be discovered, in the same way that the effects of incensole—an ingredient in frankincense—on a new brain target associated with reward (vanilloid TRP3 receptors) were.

Our seven chosen plants work on some of these signals and so support, but don't prove,

their action as mildly mind-altering plants. Although mind-altering effects are not yet part of human or lab studies (divine sage being the exception), studies on pain or sedation are common and provide clues as to which brain signals are involved, such as opioid or cannabinoid in the mind-altering mechanism. And for one of the plants, catnip, there are not surprisingly studies on pleasure-inducing behavior in cats.

PLANTS OF THE GODS

For thousands of years, people have used mind-altering plants to change their perspective, provide insights and lift their mood. We all occasionally feel the need to escape reality, and there is science to show that plants that alter perspective may indeed improve our general outlook. But recreational use, as opposed to laboratory or ritual use, can be hazardous with some of the more potent psychedelic plants. So information on how all these plants work, and can be used safely, is essential. Dilston Physic Garden plays its part in developing this knowledge, with workshops on safe mind-altering plants. One of our most popular workshops takes its name from the fascinating book, *Plants of the Gods*, by the ethnobotanist Richard Schultes and chemist Albert Hoffman. Hoffman synthesized LSD while working for the chemical company Sandoz in Switzerland, and when he tried his newly made chemical he described the experience as similar to taking magic mushrooms (*Psilocybe* spp.), which contain a similar chemical. At this point the worlds of plant and chemical highs converged.

ON THE HIT LIST

The most potent plant in our selection is divine sage (*Salvia divinorum*), which is used by Mexican and South American shamans who regard it as one of the safest for novices. This is the only plant in our selection that has been analyzed scientifically for psychedelic effects in humans. The other plants in our selection are backed by study of their active chemicals in the lab. These plants include familiar citrus fruits, frankincense, and others that are less familiar like catnip, wild lettuce, and mugwort. Natural cannabis, kava, hop, and St. John's wort also sit in the category of gentle, safe uplift balms.

Dose information is based on herbal medical use. We recommend starting at the lowest dose for the herbal medical use and noting concomitant disease and drug contraindications. Plants are listed in order

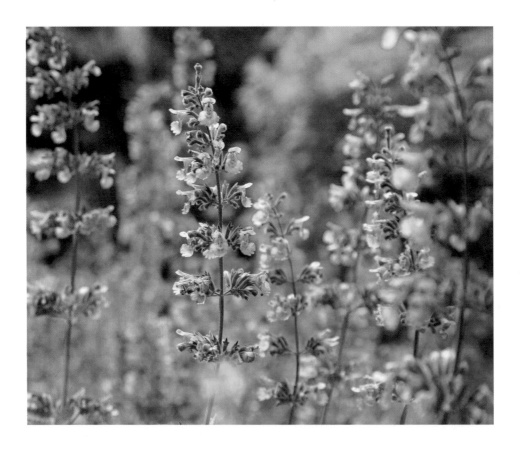

of mildest to strongest—citrus, frankincense, mugwort, catnip, wormwood, wild lettuce, and divine sage.

MORE POTENT MIND-ALTERING PLANTS

Other mind-altering plants backed by traditional use and some scientific study, like betel nut (*Areca catechu*), khat (*Catha edulis*), and peyote cactus (*Lophophora williamsii*), are more potent and illegal in some parts of the world. Synthetic illegal highs are made from these plants by extracting, synthesizing, or modifying a single chemical to produce effects much more powerful than the natural plant.

The flowering African shrub khat (*Catha edulis*) is a potent mind-altering plant that contains alkaloids related to amphetamine. Widely used in African countries, khat has recently been made illegal in most other parts of the world because, though it has clinical pain-relieving effects and is a mild euphoric stimulant used socially for millenia, it is habit forming, and overindulgence has led to misuse within communities, as well as to the production of potent synthetic derivative chemicals.

Other more potent amphetamine-like plant highs come from the Mexican mescaline-containing peyote cactus (*Lophophora*

Below: Familiar garden plants *Hypericum perforatum* (St. John's wort) and *Nepeta cataria* (catmint), **opposite,** are both gentle, safe "uplift balms."

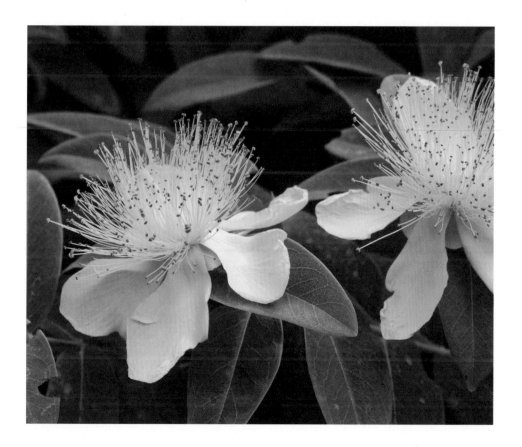

williamsii), used widely by Native Americans, and the asarone-containing sweet flag (*Acorus calamus*), which is euphoric and shown to be antidepressive and sedative in the lab. Both plants at higher doses cause hallucinations—a common feature of stronger mind-altering plants.

Nutmeg (*Myristica fragrans*) is another plant used (and abused) recreationally as a high. It's a plant medicine in Indonesia with neuroprotective and memory enhancing effects in lab studies. Its active constituent (*myristicin*)—present to a lesser extent in basil, parsley, and carrot—at high doses triggers unpleasant experiences and can produce psychosis.

Kratom (*Mitragyna speciosa*), the tropical tree in the coffee family, is an herbal medicine long used in small doses as a leaf tea to combat fatigue and improve work productivity among farm populations in Southeast Asia. It works on the same brain opiate system as divine sage and though it doesn't contain opiates, at higher doses it has opiate-like (sleep- and pain-relieving) effects. Though it's banned in many countries, a recent attempted ban in the US provoked uproar and the ban was withdrawn on account of the plant's efficacy and commonly accepted role in pain relief.

A plant with practically no science to back its psychoactive use is broom (*Cytisus scoparius*). The leaves and flower were once smoked by witches to help them "fly," and the closely related dyer's greenweed (*Genista tinctoria*), also called genista broom, is used ritualistically as a psychedelic plant in shamanic cultures in, for example, northern Mexico. Apart from their containing the alkaloid cytisine, related to nicotine, neuroscientific data is still lacking for both plants.

MIND-ALTERING BRAIN STATES AND ALTERED NEURONAL NETWORKS

Psilocybin, in magic mushrooms (*Psilocybe* spp.), boosts serotonin brain signals and improves mood in psychologically healthy volunteers. A single dose (in controlled medical circumstances) brings about profound changes, helping people to find new meaning in life. Psilocybin and other mind-altering alkaloids (tryptamines) such as dimethyltryptamine (DMT) in *Psychotria viridis* (an ingredient in ayahuasca) and ibogaine in *Tabernanthe iboga* act on the mood-boosting serotonin signal and help in psychiatric disorders and addiction. Emerging science shows they alter consciousness as they stimulate new neuronal pathways connecting areas of the brain not normally interactive. Professor Anil Seth, of the Sackler Center for Consciousness Science at the University of Sussex, concludes that the alkaloids enable the brain to reach a higher state of consciousness through electrical activity that is less integrated than during normal wakefulness.

Opposite: *Citrus × paradisi* (grapefruit), which originated in Barbados and is thought to be a cross between *C. sinensis* (orange) and *C. maxima* (pomelo), is one of many hybrid citrus fruits.

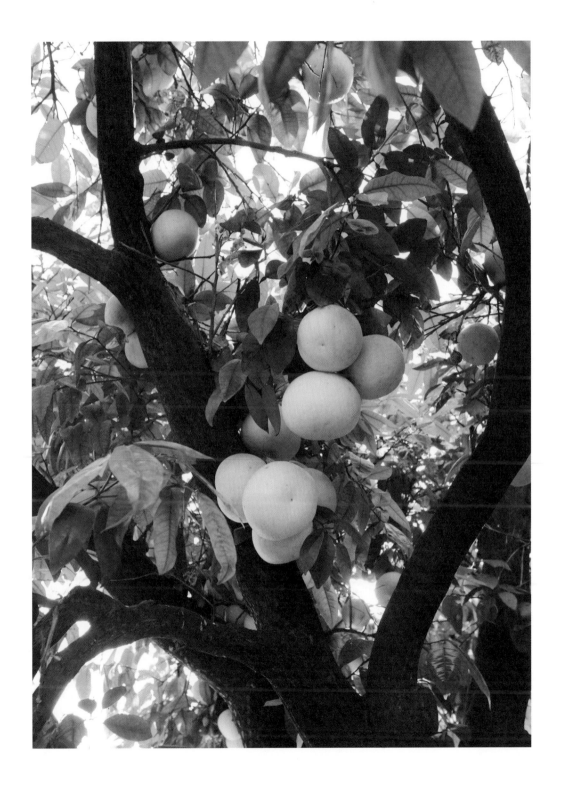

CITRUS FRUITS

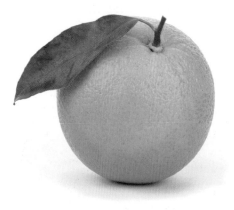

With positive effects of citrus fruits on the brain already well established, the discovery that some citrus species contain dimethyltryptamine (DMT), a potent mind-altering chemical, raises interesting questions about the feel-good effects of oranges and lemons. Neroli (bergamot flowers) and lemon are used in aromatherapy to reduce anxiety and insomnia. Many people remark on their uplifting effects, and some claim the citrus oils induce highs (but not hallucinations).

ABOUT THE PLANTS: The edible fruits such as oranges, lemons, limes, and grapefruit need no introduction, while bergamot in the same family is known for flavoring Earl Grey tea.

HISTORY AND FOLKLORE: The ancient Greeks believed that lemon leaves under the pillow induced sweet dreams, and the Spanish assign many medicinal uses to lemon. The large Indian fruit *Citrus medica* is given in Buddhist offerings. Grapefruit (*Citrus × paradisi*) originated in Barbados, where it was originally known as "forbidden fruit."

WHAT SCIENTISTS SAY

In humans: Fruit extracts, their flavonoids (such as apigenin), and their essential oils have been investigated. Clinical studies show they enhance blood flow to the brain and reduce risk of stroke and Parkinson's disease. There is increasing evidence for improving cognition.

In the lab: Extracts and their ingredients (such as naringen and hesperidin) promote new neurone connections (neuroplasticity) and are neuroprotective in different models including those associated with Alzheimer's. Various citrus species or their chemical ingredients (terpenes and flavonoids) show positive effects for pleasure (dopamine), contentment (serotonin), calming (GABA), and memory (acetylcholine) signals. Citrus chemicals have been speculated to counter any intoxicating effects of medicinal cannabis.

KEY INGREDIENTS: DMT and flavonoids such as quercetin, nobiletin, naringen, and hesperiden. Limonene, which is sedative, and citral, which has effects on memory in lab models—both affect the brain's reward and contentment signal (dopamine and serotonin). Lemon peel essential oil boosts the memory signal acetylcholine and contains similar chemicals to those in Spanish sage (*Salvia lavandulaefolia*) that have this effect.

HOW TO TAKE IT: Fresh fruit, juice or tea made with sliced fruit (especially good with fresh ginger and turmeric, which makes the DMT more effective), marmalades, and use of the essential oils such as citrus spray, which must be diluted on the skin. There are no rules on the maximum dose of fruit and juices, only on the maximum amount of certain essential oils for skin or massage as some are phototoxic:

bergamot (0.4%), lemon (2%), lime (0.7%) and grapefruit (4%).

SAFETY: Grapefruit in particular, but also some other citrus fruits, contain chemicals (furanocoumarins) that interfere with the inactivation of many drugs. They inhibit an enzyme (cytochrome P450 3A4) and so prolong or intensify drug effects with dangerous consequences. Caution for essential oils in skin allergies and with regard to phototoxicity (see "How to take it"). Legality is not an issue, despite some claims that the DMT content of citrus crops could be a source of the illegal or controlled chemical drug DMT.

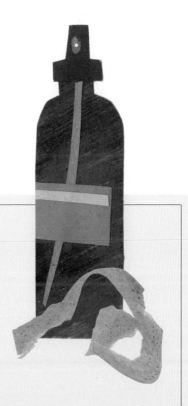

Citrus high spray

The wonderfully aromatic oils from the citrus family make an uplifting spray for wrist and neck. The steam-distilled essential oils are more concentrated, but choosing a mix from limes and lemons to exotics such as balady citron and Buddha's hand is an interesting way to make your own oil; infuse the washed and grated peel in a base oil such as coconut. Lemon scents from noncitrus plants such as lemon balm can be added to enhance the aroma.

Our favorite citrus spray is made using equal amounts of lemon, orange, mandarin, and the noncitrus but uplifting essential oil of may chang (*Itsea cubeba*). For a light, nonoily spray, simply add drops (not more than 1% total) of the essential oil to a perfumer's alcohol to disperse them, mix, and place in dark spray glass bottles. The shelf life of citrus essential oils is shorter than others and some, such as bergamot and expressed lime, can cause skin irritation and toxicity in sunlight and should not be used.

Boswellia sacra, B. serrata

FRANKINCENSE

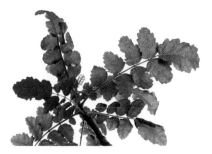

The resin from this tree provides the most widely used incense for religious and ritualistic gatherings. Its delightful aroma and ability to relieve anxiety and depression may account for feelings of being high.

ABOUT THE PLANT: A tree reaching 15 feet (4.5 m) and bearing tangled branches with the leaves clustered at the end of them, *Boswellia sacra* is native to Ethiopia, Somalia, Yemen, and Oman. It is widely found in mountainous woodland and capable of growing on bare rock. The resin, called frankincense or olibanum, is taken from many of the twenty-plus *Boswellia* species, chiefly *B. sacra*. The papery bark is slashed and the resin is allowed to dry, forming "tears" of brittle, translucent, yellowish resin collected all year. It has a spicy, lemony, and peppery aroma.

HISTORY AND FOLKLORE: Frankincense is derived from the Old French *franc encens* which means high-quality incense. It has been exported for thousands of years for use in Christian, Jewish, and other religious and spiritual gatherings—3,000-year-old frankincense was found in Tutankhamun's tomb, and the Catholic church today is a major consumer. In Ayurvedic medicine it's called *sallaki*, and among its

uses, those relating to the nervous system include stimulant, analgesic, and a remedy for emotional, psychological problems, and nervous disorders. It's said to enhance the experience of worship, and is also used as an aid to meditation to induce feelings of mental peace, satisfaction, and relaxation. It is used by some recreationally as an herbal high.

WHAT SCIENTISTS SAY

In humans: *B. serrata* is the most examined species, and massage with the essential oil (with bergamot and lavender) reduces anxiety and depression. Frankincense shows some clinical cognitive-enhancing effects and lowers cerebral edema. It's considered a safer anti-inflammatory than corticosteroids in clinical trials for osteroarthritis.

In the lab: The incense ingredient incensole acetate activates proteins in the brain via the vanilloid signal (TRPV3 receptor), which is speculated to be involved in the emotional reward response and which, in the skin, is associated with feelings of warmth. This is the first study (in 2008) to help explain emotional, and possibly also spiritual, effects of the resin. In lab models, frankincense and boswellic acid are also neuroprotective, promote growth and branching of brain cell processes that connect to other cells, improve memory in young and old models, and reduce depressive behaviors.

KEY INGREDIENTS: For analgesia and anti-depressive effects, the key active ingredients in frankincens are thought to be the terpene boswellic acids and incensole acetate. The resin is made up of up to 10% essential oil and its major ingredient is alpha-pinene. This chemical (present to varying degrees in a number of essential oils) has calming effects (GABA and glutamate modulation) and memory (acetylcholine) enhancing effects, as well as antidepressant (monoaminerigic) actions—boosting mood (serotonin), reward (dopamine) and fight or flight (noradrenaline) signals.

HOW TO TAKE IT: Capsules of resin or resin extract are commonly used. Fresh or dried resin can be consumed, and dried, burned, and inhaled as incense (using charcoal to help it burn). Frankincense essential oil is used in aromatherapy.

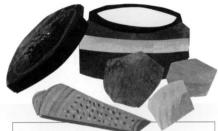

Frankincense face cream

To make this delightful face cream use a commercial face lotion, ideally organic or at least with minimal nonnatural ingredients, as a base. Mix in pure frankincense essential oil, the proportion of oil not exceeding 1%—you are likely to use generous amounts of this face cream so the frankincense dose will be sufficient to enter the system. If you can find pure organic frankincense resin, finely grate a little into the mix. Then, after mixing, put the cream in dark jars and add an attractive label. The cream seems to keep forever—several years for ours so far.

SAFETY: No side effects or contraindications reported. May cause allergic reaction. European Pharmacopoeia states extract must contain 1% of two types of boswellic acids. There are no legal restrictions to date. Rumors that church incense will be banned under the new UK legislation on legal highs and psychoactive substances have yet to be confirmed.

Artemisia vulgaris

MUGWORT

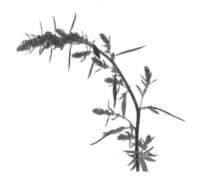

Mugwort is famous for its presence in ancient Celtic rituals, and the very few records of druid culture indicate ceremonial use. It's one of the plants that fascinates visitors to Dilston Physic Garden because of its unusual name and records in folklore of its effect on dreams.

ABOUT THE PLANT: It has spiked green leaves, silvery and hairy underneath, and clusters of small reddish flowerheads. Native to Asia, North Africa, and Europe, it can reach up to 6 feet (1.8 m). Chinese mugwort (*A. argyi* and *A. verlotorum*) grows as well as *A. vulgaris* in temperate regions and has an even more alluring aroma and flavor for tea.

HISTORY AND FOLKLORE: Also called wild wormwood or witches herb, in ancient Celtic rituals *A. vulgaris* was used to enhance spiritual states of mind, and in Saxon times it was one of the nine sacred herbs that were believed to protect against infection. Roman soldiers used to stuff their sandals with mugwort to help them march longer, implying more potent high effects. In China, mugwort has been valued for millennia and is the ingredient used in the alternative therapy moxibustion (where stimulation with heat from a stick of mugwort is used at acupuncture points). Mugwort has been traditionally used as an analgesic, sedative, hypertensive, hypnotic, for tremor in Parkinson's disease, and by British physicians for epilepsy in the early nineteenth century. Mild euphoric cannabis-like highs are reported (Mexican mugwort, *A. mexicana*, is used as a cannabis substitute) and subtle alterations in consciousness such as sharpening colors and clarifying meaning.

Smudging with mugwort

Native American smudging is said to clear obstructions and set the scene for sacred rituals. Wafting the aromatic smoke from a smudging stick made from dried plant, most commonly white sage (*Salvia apiana*), which has effects at the cannabinoid receptor, may have perception-shifting effects. Mugwort (the most aromatic is Chinese mugwort, *Artemisia argyi*, which grows readily in temperate zones) or any other of the plants described in this chapter can be substituted, though there needs to be a way of keeping the plant material glowing and smoking (the traditionally used plants do this naturally). The stages in our mugwort smudging are:

Pick the top stems of mugwort before flowering and hang them to dry in a cool well-ventilated room out of the sun. After two weeks, strip off the leaves and store in brown paper bags. (Alternatively, buy dried mugwort leaves.)

Mix the leaves with a little wood or bamboo charcoal, light, burn for a short while, and then gently put out the flame and allow the mix to smolder. The smoke can be wafted around using a feather or just by flapping a hand.

To follow the ritual tradition, smoke is wafted around each person's head, above, below and in the four cardinal directions (north, south, east, and west). To benefit more from the effects of mugwort, the smoke can be inhaled directly.

It's said to promote vivid and pleasant dreams and also lucid dreams where you sleep but stay aware and change your dreams to suit yourself. Volunteers in our physic garden report that after weeding the mugwort bed they feel "spaced out" and relaxed.

WHAT SCIENTISTS SAY

In humans: Mugwort moxibustion that uses acupuncture points has been studied and may be beneficial in hypertension.

In the lab: Its constituent thujone (also in common sage) has effects on sedative (GABA), memory, and attention (acetylcholine), and its psychotropic effects are potentially due to alterations in serotonin and cannabinoid signals, though it does not produce the same response as cannabis. *A. maderaspatana* increases the main memory signal (acetylcholine) by preventing its breakdown.

KEY INGREDIENTS: Contains flavonoids, tannins and bitter glycosides similar to wormwood. Essential oil contains thujone (also in wormwood), borneol, cineole, camphor and pinene, which are all present in sage and other aromatic plants. They affect various signals in the brain (memory, calming and excitatory).

HOW TO TAKE IT: Tea, fresh (3 to 5 g) or dried (2 to 3 g) per 240 ml water 3 times daily (it can be bitter). A tincture is also commonly used. It can be smoked and added to stir-fries.

SAFETY: Do not use in pregnancy. Caution in epilepsy. May cause an allergic reaction. Not for regular use. Essential oil is toxic.

Nepeta cataria and other species

CATNIP

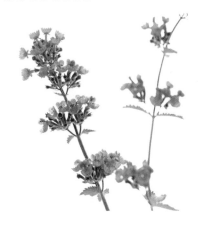

This plant is loved by cats for its pleasure-inducing effects and also by some humans, who use it as a mild and safe uplift balm.

ABOUT THE PLANT: Catmint, catwort, or field balm is a sweet mint-like aromatic plant, one of 250 species. It grows wild in northern temperate chalky regions and is cultivated for use in the pet industry. The heart-shaped leaves are whitish-green and the flowers are white, with traces of blue or lavender. It reaches up to 39 inches (1 m) and can be grown in containers—useful if you want to keep it from being flattened by cats.

HISTORY AND FOLKLORE: It was once used by those too poor to afford tea from China, who insisted it gave as much pleasure and was much more wholesome. It's been long known for its relaxing euphoric and aphrodisiac effects on both domestic and wild cats such as leopards and lynxes—the scent is similar to pheromones in male cat urine. The Egyptians thought their cats were incarnated gods and gave them catnip. It's used in traditional medicine in Europe and Asia as a relaxant, to reduce nightmares, and for migraine pain.

From its reputation as a plant loved by cats comes the saying about catnip promoting "kitty in the sky"—a play on the Beatles song "Lucy in the Sky with Diamonds," referring to LSD. However, catnip is not like LSD and though used by some as an herbal high, it's also a safe herbal medicine. Mildly mind-altering, it brings a sense of well-being known as the mellows. Some people say they experience a mild buzz and occasional hallucination, described by some as similar to a shamanic state of mind.

WHAT SCIENTISTS SAY

In humans: Iranian catnip (*N. menthoides*) has been shown to relieve anxiety, depression, and memory impairment in controlled clinical trials.

In the lab: *N. cataria* has mild sedative effects, *N. bracteata* is anticonvulsant, and a few species (such as *N. caesarea*) have been shown to have sedative and analgesic effects via brain opiate receptors—acting by a nonaddictive mechanism. Catnip affects the pleasure pathways (dopamine), is aphrodisiac and amphetamine-like. *N. menthoides* prevents morphine dependence and improves memory in lab models. Cineole-containing essential oil and also diterpenes from certain species increase the memory signal (acetylcholine) as powerfully as the prescribed drugs.

KEY INGREDIENTS: Nepetalactone acts on smell (olfactory) signals, inducing euphoria in cats (it also repels flies). Nepethalate and ursolic acid are sedative, and ursolic acid acts via the opioid signal and boosts the memory

signal. Essential oil contains citronellol and geraniol, which are calming in humans, and pulegone, which is both antianxiety and stimulant. Lemon catnip (*N. cataria* var. *citriodora*) has polyphenols—flavonoids similar to lemon balm, such as the antianxiety luteolin and apigenin, along with rosmarinic acid that also boosts the memory signal—key antioxidants and anti-inflammatories.

HOW TO TAKE IT: Tea of leaves and flowers, fresh (2 to 4 g) or dried (1 to 2 g) per 240 ml water 3 times daily are delicious. Leaf and flower also make a fine alcoholic spirit, can be smoked, burnt as a soothing and relaxing incense, and the essential oil inhaled over steam or in a room diffuser.

SAFETY: Widely considered safe as an herbal medicine with no known contraindications. Nausea at higher doses is reported. Essential oil is a possible skin sensitizer. Part of the 2016 UK Psychoactive Plant Ban, implying that the mind-altering effects of this previously legal herbal high are taken seriously. But regulation of this ornamental and safe medicinal plant growing in many gardens and sold in garden centers will be challenging, and it's legal in most other countries, including the US.

Artemisia absinthium

WORMWOOD

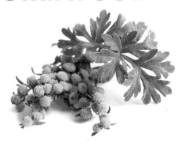

Wormwood is a plant more famous for its role in absinthe, the mind-altering "green fairy" liqueur popular with nineteenth-century artists, than for its ability to remove intestinal worms, which gives it its common name.

ABOUT THE PLANT: This elegant tall perennial in the daisy family has feathery silver-green leaves with characteristic small globular yellow flowerheads. It has a sharp, spicy scent and bitter flavor. Sweet wormwood (*A. annua*) has also been studied clinically.

HISTORY AND FOLKLORE: The legend of its mythical name is that when water and absinthe mix the green fairy (said to be lucidity of thought) is set free—dilution with water produces a whitish tinge. A symbol of sin in the Bible, wormwood was said to grow in the tracks of the serpent that crawled from the Garden of Eden. The ancient Egyptians considered it an aphrodisiac, and it's used in plant medicine today to uplift, as a restorative tonic for mental debility, and to calm nervous dispositions. The essential oil is widely used as a flavoring ingredient in liqueurs such as Pernod. Hallucinations experienced by absinthe drinkers, who notably included Van Gogh, were more probably due to the alcohol than the plant, which by itself is not now considered hallucinogenic. According to reports, effects vary from mildly sedative to inducing vivid, especially lucid, dreaming (it's in the same genus as mugwort). Wormwood's appetite-stimulating and digestive actions no doubt add to the value of the liqueur.

WHAT SCIENTISTS SAY

In humans: Studies have focused on its controlled clinical efficacy on the gut (Crohn's) and in pain relief in arthritis.

In the lab: Affects attention and memory pathways—its ingredient thujone blocks the action of nicotine (nicotinic receptor) but prevents breakdown of the memory signal (acetylcholine). Thujone is stimulatory by blocking the action of the calming signal (GABA), and affects the brain molecules that bind cannabinoids and serotonin. Wormwood is also neuroprotective and anti-inflammatory in the brain.

KEY INGREDIENTS: Contains beta-thujone, sabinyl acetate, and the calming beta-pinene. Also contains sesquiterpene lactones such as absinthin and bitter flavonoid glycosides.

HOW TO TAKE IT: Leaves, fresh (4 to 6 g) or dried (2 to 3 g) per 240 ml water 3 times daily can be used to make a bitter-tasting tea. Also smoked (dried), taken as a tincture, or as absinthe liqueur (which traditionally also contains lemon balm and hyssop)—it's well worth making your own liqueur if you grow the plant.

SAFETY: High thujone content means wormwood cannot be used in epilepsy, pregnancy, (where it's abortifacient) or aromatherapy. No other contraindications are reported. There are no restrictions today on the plant or absinthe. Like mugwort, not for regular use.

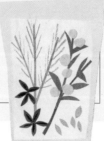

Lactuca virosa

WILD LETTUCE

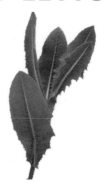

This is the plant from which the culinary salad lettuce was cultivated. Its other name, opium lettuce, is an indication of its potential use as an herbal high.

ABOUT THE PLANT: A deeply lobed broad-leaved, hollow-stemmed plant in the daisy family growing to just over 39 inches (1 m). Tiny dandelion-like yellow flowers turn to puffs of thistledown-like fluff that contain the seeds, so the plant spreads widely. It's found growing wild across Europe, and all parts contain a pungent milky white latex. Harvesting takes place before it flowers.

HISTORY AND FOLKLORE: Psychoactive properties were recorded in ancient Egyptian scripts and in the first century AD Greek physician Dioscorides wrote that its effect was similar to opium poppy (*Papaver somniferum*). This may be why wild lettuce can be mistakenly viewed as toxic even at normal doses. It became known as "lettuce opium" in the nineteenth century when physicians couldn't obtain opium and it was found to be free from opium's side effects. In plant medicine it's a sedative and hypnotic, used to calm overactivity and overstimulation in adults and children, as well as to relieve pain and to lower libido (anaphrodisiac). Garden lettuce (*Lactuca sativa*) contains similar chemicals and its stalks, with much weaker therapeutic action, are mildly euphoric and soporific. Beatrix Potter referenced this in her flopsy bunnies, who stuffed themselves with overgrown lettuces and fell asleep before getting caught by Mr. McGregor.

The dried latex, called lactucarium, was listed in the British Pharmacopoeia 1885, for use as a mild hypnotic. The mature leaves and stems of wild lettuce, dried and smoked, are said to induce mild euphoria and spaced-out states. It is reported to promote meditative, trance-like states and dreaming.

WHAT SCIENTISTS SAY

In humans: Wild lettuce has not been studied clinically due to reports showing overdose causes toxicity. *L. sativa* seed oil improves sleep and anxiety in older patients with mild to moderate anxiety and sleep difficulties. There are no classic opioid actions (such as morphine), so addiction is not a problem.

In the lab: Its ingredients sedate via the calming (GABA) pathway (a similar hypnotic effect to pentobarbital but without toxicity). They are also analgesic, increase the attention and memory chemical acetylcholine (stopping its breakdown), and have sleep control (adenosine) actions.

KEY INGREDIENTS: Effects are due to sesquiterpene lactones such as lactucin and related lactucopicrin, which are analgesic (comparable to ibuprofen) and are also found in chicory (*Cichorium intybus*).

HOW TO TAKE IT: Most efficient mode is said to be latex (dried lactucarium) as a tablet or capsule of powder (take as instructed). As the latex does not dissolve in water, teas of fresh or dried plant may not be very active compared to tinctures or smoking.

SAFETY: Safe only in recommended dose. Causes drowsiness at higher doses. Side effects include dizziness, tachycardia (rapid heartbeat), and loss of libido. As it can be used as a recreational drug, the potential is definitely there for people to take excessive amounts and this can be toxic. No contraindication reported. Not a controlled plant in most countries.

Salvia divinorum
DIVINE SAGE

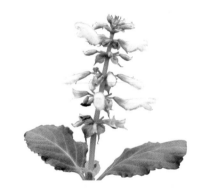

South American shamans use divine sage to alter states of consciousness as an introduction to "spirit journeys," and it's also used (and abused) recreationally round the world. The plant and its chemical are the subject of much scientific research.

ABOUT THE PLANT: A rare plant in the mint family with long, succulent stems and large, velvety, mint-like leaves, though not aromatic.

It thrives in warm climates and is best grown indoors in sunlight in temperate zones, where it rarely produces its white flowers

HISTORY AND FOLKLORE: Also known as seer's sage and holy sage, it's been used for hundreds of years as a divining tool in South America, and in healing ceremonies and medicinally by Mazatec Indians in Oaxaca, Mexico, where it is a native known as *ska Maria pastora*, meaning "leaves of the Virgin Mary, the Shepherdess." It's referred to as "magic mint" by recreational users in the West today, while the Mazatecs term it a divine inebriation. Users speak of laughing, feeling they are merging with their surroundings, and seeing interesting visions. Using the leaves at the correct dose is safe, and there's said to be a wonderful afterglow, a peaceful euphoria that lasts an hour or two. There are anecdotal reports of use in treating depression.

WHAT SCIENTISTS SAY

In humans: The plant (combusted and inhaled) provides a rapid onset and intense, unique, short-lived, and mostly pleasant experience with mild changes in visual and auditory input, and people report losing awareness of themselves and their surroundings. Though not examined in detail clinically, there's no evidence of persisting effects, and it's widely believed to have low addictive potential and low toxicity. Effects are blocked by the drug naloxone, which blocks the pain (opioid) pathway. *S. divinorum* is currently being explored for effects that may help in treating depression. Studies on the active constituent (salvinorin A, not recommended because of potency) indicate very rapid effects (within minutes of inhalation) and similar changes in sensory perception, as with the whole plant.

In the lab: Salvinorin A (around 0.2 percent of plant) acts on the same opioid signal (kappa) in the brain as opium does. This is different from the one that causes addiction (another type, mu), and it's therefore being explored as a treatment for drug addiction. Kappa is concentrated in an area of the brain (the claustrum) that's highly connected to many cells of the cerebral cortex (linked to higher intelligence), and has been implicated in consciousness itself. Salvinorin A also affects reward (dopamine) signals and is sedative, antianxiety, antidepressant and impairs learning and memory in lab models.

KEY INGREDIENTS: Diterpenes called salvinorins, with studies concentrated on salvinorin A a volatile psychoactive terpene, are aiding the understanding of opioid signals (kappa receptors).

HOW TO TAKE IT: Traditionally a "quid" (a portion of leaves) is chewed like tobacco and not swallowed, keeping saliva in the mouth for as long as possible. It is important to get the dose right, starting at a lower dose and not to overdose. A quantity of 7 g, about 1 to 2 large fresh leaves (or 3 to 8 g dried leaves) is recommended, and effects can last for two hours. The leaves are bitter though and people often inhale the smoke or smoke them instead, where the mind-altering effect is said to be more acute.

SAFETY: Considered safe at appropriate dose. As our most potent consciousness-expanding plant, it can be associated with abuse and, at high doses, negative psychological effects, but no more so than cannabis and alcohol. Some recommend being with a "sitter" in case of feelings of disorientation. Not to be mixed with alcohol. Caution with cardiovascular conditions—can increase heart rate. Do not use the pure chemical salvinorin A recreationally since it is dangerous due to its acute potency. *S. divinorum* should not be taken by vulnerable individuals or by those with psychological/psychiatric conditions unless under supervision. Legal in most countries at present but controls are being introduced. This plant may follow the path of cannabis, which was banned on account of the use of concentrated chemicals derived from it and species bred for the higher pyschoactive ingredients, but now traditionally used species with natural ratios of ingredients are being reinstated in some places.

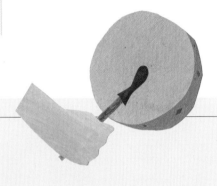

Shamanic journeys by the bonfire

Shamanic practices are primarily aimed at healing. They involve journeying to what is perceived as the spirit world for guidance using the intuitive, subconscious, and creative mind. A practice familiar to Westerners is the Amazonian shamanic rituals using the potent hallucinogenic ayahuasca plant mix.

One shamanic journeying path we find intriguing, safe, and satisfying is to follow a drumbeat with guiding words for the journey, led by a shamanic practitioner. You can gather round a bonfire and perhaps sip a tea or spirit made from a plant in this chapter. Here's a rough guide:

Sit comfortably for about 20 minutes as the drum beats slowly.

Be guided into an "underworld" of delightful scenery, sounds, and sights by visualizing the process of walking in the open countryside and then entering a tunnel (not unlike the Alice in Wonderland white rabbit experience).

Visualize looking for and "meeting" your personal spirit guide, usually an animal, and listening to what this being has to say to you.

Visualize traveling back to where you are sitting as the drumbeat speeds up and then stops.

Reflect on your experience and share it with the group if you like.

As with any new mental experience, a shamanic journey may uncover the negative as well as positive, so it is best to have a trained professional on hand for at least the first few times. While there are many who call themselves shamans, the title strictly belongs to those trained for a lifetime by a traditional shaman—others are "shamanic practitioners" and it's worth checking out their reputation.

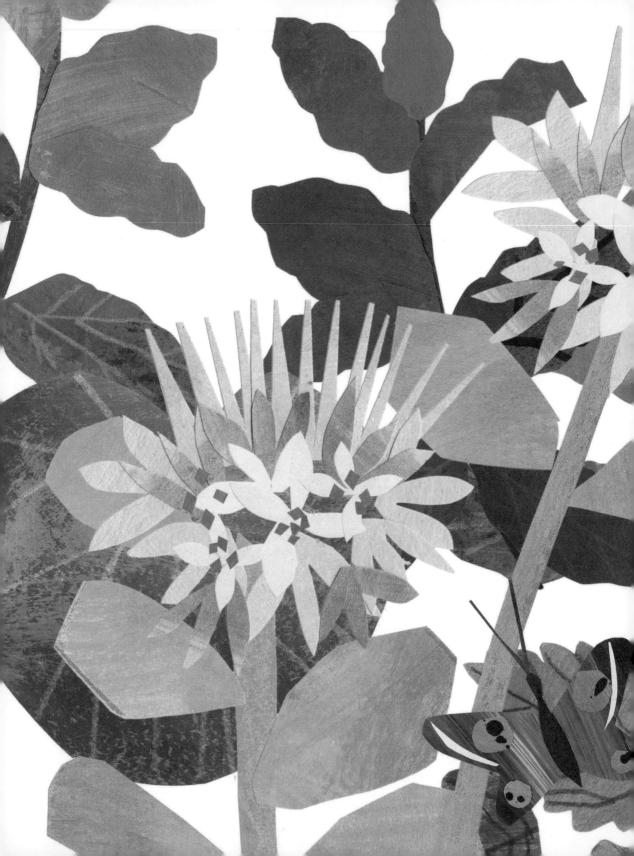

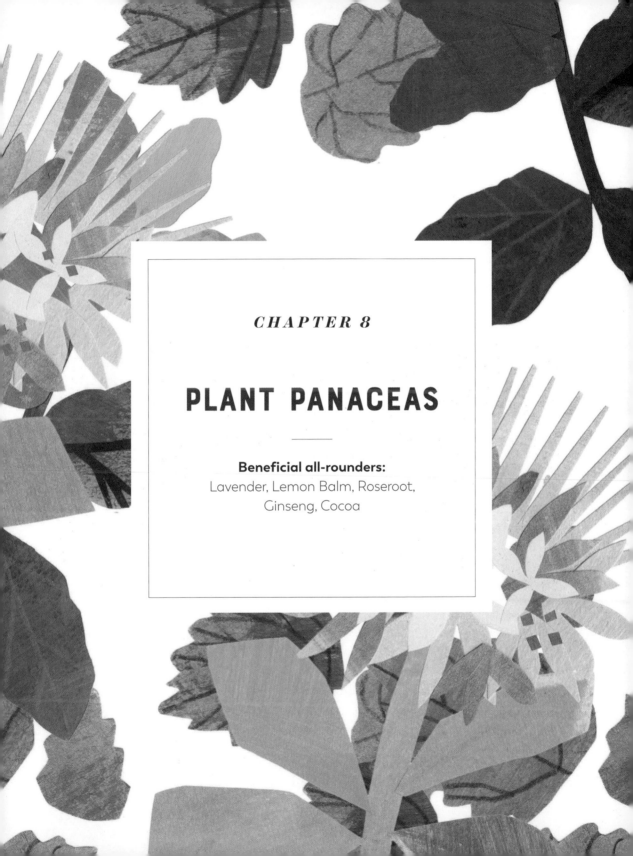

CHAPTER 8

PLANT PANACEAS

Beneficial all-rounders:
Lavender, Lemon Balm, Roseroot,
Ginseng, Cocoa

How have we got to Chapter 8 with no mention of lavender or ginseng, two of the best-known plants for medicinal qualities? These and other important plants such as roseroot are actually front-runner brain balms, with wide-ranging benefits—almost panaceas for mood and mind—and they have been reserved for this final chapter.

Lavender is a good example of a plant with many benefits—it promotes sleep, relieves pain, and may even improve memory, while roseroot eases anxiety, low mood, and fatigue. The five panacea balms in this chapter represent some of the most effective plants available for treating a wide range of common conditions of the mind and brain.

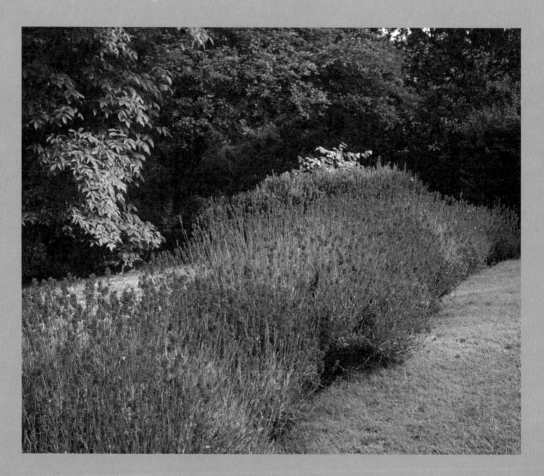

ONE PLANT, SEVERAL ACTIONS

Medical herbalists recognize that medicinal plants work on more than one symptom or system and this makes sense scientifically—first because each plant contains more than one active ingredient that can target different systems, and second because the health of one part of the body is affected by other parts, with links between heart and mind an obvious example.

The brain is not divided into boxes—it is the most highly connected living system, each function affected by others. This is why depression or sleep deprivation can impair cognitive function, and stress or anxiety can interfere with memory or increase the feeling of pain.

Hawthorn for health

Hawthorn (*Crataegus species*) clinically reduces cardiovascular risk factors such as hypertension, high cholesterol, and atherosclerosis, while increasing exercise tolerance and lowering cardiac oxygen consumption, shortness of breath, and fatigue. Hawthorn's different bioactive compounds are responsible for its multiple actions—the flavonoid hyperoside increases coronary flow, oleanolic acid inhibits ACE activity and lowers cholesterol, proanthocyanidins are vasodilatory, and epicatechin has cardioprotective effects.

POLYPHARMACOLOGY

Using different drugs to treat a range of symptoms, and targeting them to the individual, is increasingly common in mainstream medicine. For example, a person's heart condition could be treated with one drug to lower blood pressure and another to thin the blood. Single-chemical drugs tend to target specific symptoms and so are used together to help set a system right. This is where medicinal plants can step in, with the different chemicals in one plant working synergistically, with fewer side effects, to have more than one effect. One such example is hawthorn, with its red berry (haw) containing several bioactive compounds, shown in clinical trials to safely and significantly help treat heart failure by a number of different actions. And while lab studies show how such different bioactive chemicals in any one plant act on different systems in the body and brain to produce a holistic effect, testing single plant chemicals in humans can't be done without huge investment in testing safety and dose.

As well as multiple chemicals in one plant working together (polypharmacology), combinations of plants given as one single medicine are used in herbal medicine—a combination of sage, rosemary, and lemon balm for example improves memory. But our panacea balms are single plants that affect the many areas of mental well-being considered in the first seven chapters.

Opposite: *Lavandula officinalis* (lavender) has a wide-ranging set of benefits for mind and brain.

POTENTIAL PLANT PANACEAS

Potential plant panaceas for the future are ashwagandha and kava-kava, calming balms that also improve memory and stamina and are antiaging; sage, the cognition balm, that also calms, improves mood, and reduces fatigue; and nigella, a cognition balm that reduces anxiety and enhances mood as well as having other effects on the body.

FIVE ALL-ROUNDER BALMS

Our five exceptional plant panaceas share four or more of the calm, memory, mood, sleep, pain, or energy balm functions, backed by human clinical trials and lab science. We start with two aromatics in the European mint family, lavender and lemon balm, the latter being a focus of much of our university research for effects on mood and memory. They are followed by the striking arctic roseroot, renowned for helping with fatigue but with other cognitive benefits—and a plant we appreciate since it loves our cooler Northumbrian climate. Then comes the great energizer ginseng from China, often billed as the most famous of all medicinal plants, and cocoa from South America, the only all-rounder known to have mind-expanding qualities.

ALL ROUND THE BODY

The brain depends on controlled oxygen and energy supplies more than any other body part; heart, gut, and metabolic functions (to mention a few) are intimately involved. The five plant panaceas have effects on the body likely to affect brain function. Lavender's lab studies indicate beneficial blood glucose-controlling effects and protection against bacterial-induced colitis. Lemon balm improves blood vessel function and blood lipid profiles, and lowers heart palpitations. Roseroot improves aerobic

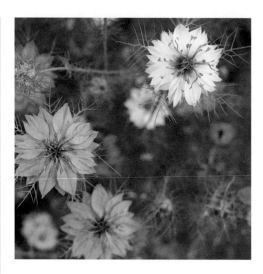

Above: *Nigella sativa* (nigella) is a cognition balm that reduces anxiety and enhances mood.
Opposite: *Melissa officinalis* (lemon balm) is one of our five exceptional plant panaceas.

exercise performance, relieves ischaemic heart disease symptoms, and in a meta-analysis improves cardiac function in angina patients and regulates blood lipid and glycogen. Our last two panacea balms, ginseng and cocoa, have what plant medicine calls "adaptogenic" properties—they increase resistance to stress—and some controlled trials show ginseng improves cardiac function, controls blood glucose, and has other effects on aging, immunity, and cancer. Finally, cocoa lowers blood pressure and risk of heart disease as well as stroke, and may even improve metabolic function (regulating blood glucose). Tempting as it may be to make these connections, there is not yet evidence directly linking these bodily effects with brain benefits.

MELISSA OFFICINALIS, THE ULTIMATE BALM

Lemon balm (*Melissa officinalis*) took us by surprise in trials we conducted—it worked to improve memory in young people, acted as

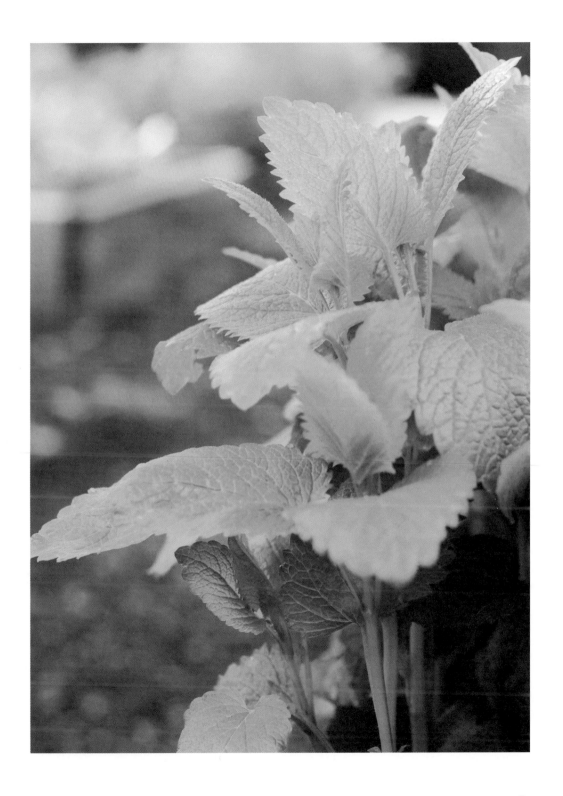

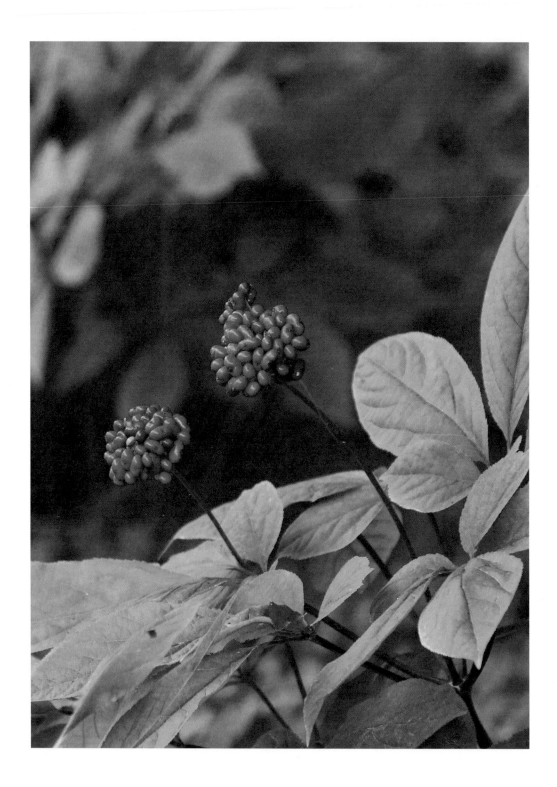

YOUR BRAIN ON PLANTS

a calming agent in old people, and in the last trial improved the quality of life in people with dementia. Following those trials we learned others had shown that lemon balm also relieves pain and helps sleep. It has active terpene and phenolic ingredients, and the team at Durham University continues its work to pin down the calming action to one chemical in lab experiments, seeing how the plant extract or constituent chemicals reduce electrical impulses in nerve cells. Whether any one chemical will account for the different actions of lemon balm remains to be seen—but the chemical drug aspirin is a reminder that one simple molecule can achieve a great many different health benefits.

Opposite: *Panax quinquefolius* (ginseng) and *Theobroma cacao* (cocoa) **below** both make it into our top five plant panaceas.

SKEPTICAL IN THE WEST

While ginseng stands out as a plant revered in traditional Chinese medicine and is the subject of many scientific studies, both in trials in humans and in the lab, there is still skepticism from Western reviewers regarding the evidence. This tends to leave people with the option of taking an Eastern or Western view. Trying to bridge this gap would need another book, but ginseng is a prime example of a theme that runs through many of our plant profiles: that evidence from human studies, while supporting traditional uses, often does not yet satisfy the strict criteria on quality and quantity for drug trials. However, without resources, which are hard to come by for plant medicines that can't be patented, the studies that exist are the best evidence yet, alongside their centuries-old traditional evidence base.

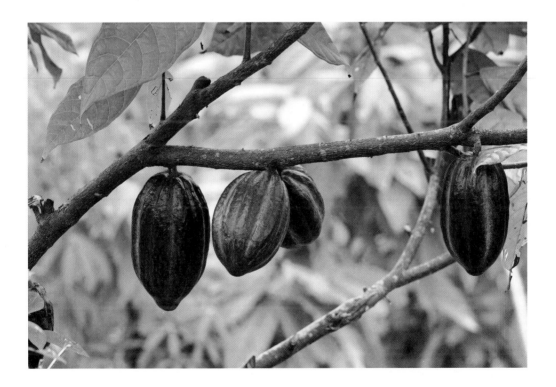

Lavandula officinalis syn. *L. angustifolia*

LAVENDER

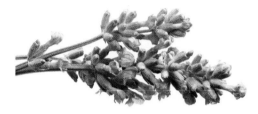

One of the most famous European medicinal plants and the most used essential oil, lavender has a wide range of benefits for the brain and mind, from calming and inducing sleep to relieving depression and pain.

ABOUT THE PLANT: Lavender is an evergreen 39 inches (1 m) perennial woody shrub from the Mediterranean that likes well-drained soil and sunny slopes. The scent of both its narrow silvery-green leaves and purplish-blue flowers is crisp, clean, floral, and sweet. It's spectacular grown in lavender farms, where swathes of intense color blanket the ground in midsummer. The medicinal value of the numerous cultivars is unknown.

HISTORY AND FOLKLORE: It's been recorded since ancient times for health benefits and use as perfume. Tutankhamun's tomb contained traces of still-fragrant lavender, and the Romans named the plant after its use in their bathing rituals. Greek physician Dioscorides wrote that lavender taken internally relieves indigestion, sore throats, and headaches, and externally cleans wounds. Its use in World War II to heal wounds led to the practice of aromatherapy. Sixteenth-century English herbalist John Parkinson wrote lavender was "especially good use for all griefes and paines of the head and brain" and medical herbalists today use lavender for stress-induced headaches, migraines, earaches, neuralgia, other bodily benefits, and for all the uses now verified scientifically.

WHAT SCIENTISTS SAY

In humans: In controlled trials, lavender promoted calm and reduced anxiety and related restlessness in several settings, and the essential oil capsules were well tolerated, comparable to conventional drugs for anxiety. Also relieves anxiety before and after surgery and during dental treatment. In pregnancy, depression, and hospice patients it relieves depression and improves well-being.

When given with imipramine, a drug for depression, lavender improved the benefits compared to the drug on its own. In a separate study it was found comparable to the SSRI paroxetine for depression. Social issues can be linked to depression, and lavender increased interpersonal trust (in a game situation) compared to peppermint and promoted infant bonding in new mothers (this effect is short-term).

For sleep Lavender capsules improve sleep, and inhalation of lavender improves sleep in coronary intensive care and cancer patients in controlled trials, as well as improving self-rated sleep quality and energy in students with sleep problems. It also reduces restless leg syndrome.

For memory In pilot trials lavender inhalation reduced working memory when inhaled in normal circumstances, but after stress conditions it improved working memory.

For pain The essential oil relieved headache, joint, carpal tunnel, dysmenorrhoea, and pain during and post surgery, and in muscle spasm in a review of trials. Also topically treats bruises, burns, and wounds.

In the lab: Essential oil or its individual chemicals (such as linalool) block the excitatory (glutamate) neurotransmitter and act on mood-lifting (serotonin and dopamine) signals. These effects are also seen following inhalation. Lab studies also show action on calcium channels and confirm antidepressant, sedative, pain-relieving, anti-inflammatory and memory-improving effects, as well as being antiaging and protective in memory models.

KEY INGREDIENTS: Volatile (essential) oil contains more than 40 constituents, the main anxiety-relieving chemicals are the terpenes linalool and its ester linalyl acetate (which are also present in other aromatic plants and in citrus fruits). Also contains the memory-boosting cineole and camphor shown in lab studies. Composition of essential oil varies depending on many factors but should contain 25 to 38 percent linalool, 25 to 45 percent linalyl acetate and 0.3 to 1.5 percent cineole.

HOW TO TAKE IT: Use the essential oil in aromatherapy by putting 3 to 4 undiluted drops directly on a pillow, clothing, tissue, or in the bath. Flowers are also used to make teas and tinctures, and also in culinary dishes and drinks—a lavender syrup or vodka made with the essential oil can be added to a champagne cocktail.

SAFETY: Lavender is one of the safest plants and its essential oil can be applied undiluted, though can occasionally cause skin irritation. May exacerbate sedative or anticonvulsant drugs, and because of estrogenic properties, not recommended in young males. There are hazards associated with taking the attractive species French lavender (*L. stoechas*) internally, with reports of toxicity in children.

Lavender—an alternative to conventional drugs for anxiety?

Trials of lavender essential oil to calm are numerous and a standardized capsulated essential oil called Silexan has recently been tested in controlled trials led by the Medical University of Vienna, Austria. Lavender (silexan) was found comparable to the benzodiazepine lorazepam (in a multicenter placebo-controlled trial in 450 people) and to the antidepressant (SSRI) paroxetine (in a randomized, double-blind, placebo-controlled trial in 539 adults). The safety of silexan has been demonstrated, and as well as inducing calm it also improves sleep and depression and is without side effects, drug interactions, or dependency. And with proven dose-dependent effects this is a classic example of how using standardized extracts of plants in trial settings produces consistent data.

Forest bathing

People have long understood the health benefits of walking in nature. The wonderfully-named *Shinrin-yoku*, or "forest bathing," is standard preventative medicine in Japan. Field experiments conducted across twenty-four forests in Japan showed that levels of the stress hormone cortisol decreased in test subjects after a walk in the forest, when compared with a control group of subjects who engaged in walks within the city. Overexposure to cortisol and other stress hormones can lead to memory and concentration impairment, so a walk in the woods can be a good way to combat these problems.

Try walking silently among trees, enjoying the aromas that stimulate and soothe and tuning in to the sounds of the forest. As you encounter individual specimens such as oak, rowan, yew, manuka, holly, and banyan, remember that they were once regarded as sacred by earlier civilizations. Marvel at their longevity—some trees live for thousands of years—and wonder at their solid trunks that reach from deep in the earth to high in the sky.

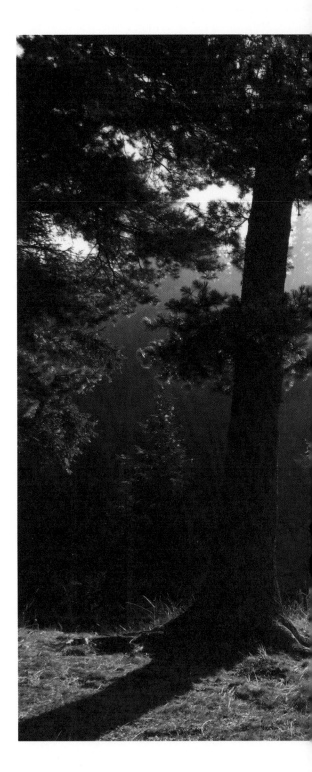

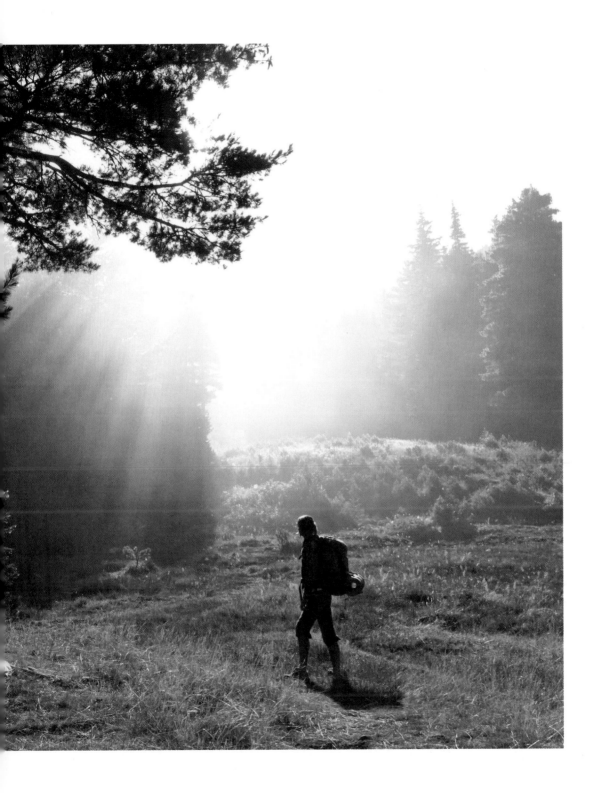

Melissa officinalis

LEMON BALM

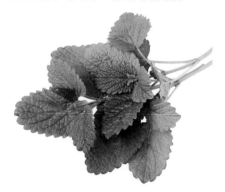

This modest plant, also known as melissa, offers a delightful lemony aroma and flavor as well as significant benefits for anxiety, mood, memory, sleep, and pain. It has a long-standing reputation as a plant for relaxation and enhancing cognition

ABOUT THE PLANT: A member of the mint family, this native to southern Europe, northern Africa, and West Asia is a low, bushy perennial with heart-shaped leaves and tiny white flowers. Growing and spreading almost anywhere temperate, it's hardy, though the leaves usually die back in winter. It's not ideal as a potted plant, but the equally aromatic lemon verbena (*Aloysia citrodora*) thrives in a pot and has similar chemicals and effects.

HISTORY AND FOLKLORE: Lemon balm has long been used by beekeepers to calm their bees. Sixteenth-century English herbalist Gerard claimed that it "causeth the Bees to stick together and causeth others to come unto them." According to *The London Dispensary* of 1696, "An essence of Balm, given in Canary wine, every morning will renew youth, strengthen the brain, relieve languishing

nature and prevent baldness" and if used regularly it was thought to promote long life. Seventeenth-century herbalist John Evelyn said "Balm is sovereign for the brain, strengthening the memory and powerfully chasing away melancholy." Medical herbalists today use lemon balm as a mild sedative to reduce panic, palpitations, restlessness, mild depression, and sleeplessness, and for its relaxing and uplifting properties, as well as for digestive problems caused by anxiety (indigestion, bloating, colic), and more. In Western herbal medicine it is often used in combination with valerian.

WHAT SCIENTISTS SAY

In humans: For calming and blues-busting
Controlled trials support lemon balm's ability to improve mood and reduce anxiety, palpitations, and agitation, and in some trials in people with dementia where it also improves quality of life, to calm young people, and to relieve premenstrual tension and associated psychological symptoms in teenage girls. In combination with valerian it reduced hyperactivity, concentration difficulties, and impulsiveness in observational trials in primary school children.

For memory It improves cognitive processing, memory, and attention in healthy adults and in Alzheimer's in controlled trials.

For sleep Lemon balm, again with valerian, relieved sleep disorders in a multicenter trial in menopausal women, in an observational study in children, and in a pilot study.

For pain With fennel and chamomile, lemon balm relieved pain, headache, and colic in a controlled trial in 88 infants.

In the lab: Extracts increase the action of the brain calming signal (GABA) and extracts and chemicals (such as citronellal) are antispasmodic, sedative, and anxiety relieving. Lemon balm relieves depression, accelerates sleep onset, and prolongs sleep time in lab models, where effects are enhanced when combined with lavender (*Lavandula officinalis*). It acts on other brain systems including the one for attention and memory (muscarinic and nicotinic receptors for acetylcholine), and is also analgesic (rosmarinic acid and eugenol), neuroprotective, antiarrhythmic, and reduces inflammation, oxidation, and hyperlipidemia.

KEY INGREDIENTS: Essential oil containing sedative terpenes such as citronelal (also analgesic), neral, and geranial—which are known together as citral and are also found in citrus fruit, especially the peel, and in other aromatic plants such as lemongrass (*Cymbopogon citratus*), lemon verbena, and the Australian sweet verbena tree (*Backhousia citriodora*). Citronellal and citral are both responsible for the lemony flavor. The oil also contains caryophyllene oxide and the calming linalool and geraniol. Key polyphenols such as rosmarinic and caffeic acids and flavonoids such as luteolin are also important.

Lemonbalmade

Per 1 quart (1 L) bottle
Use about 6 handfuls fresh lemon balm
 (*Melissa officinalis*) leaves
2 tablespoons honey (or to taste)
2 lemons
Sparkling water, to serve

Pick fresh unblemished leaves on a sunny morning—the best are at the growing tips of the plant before it flowers. Put them in a large teapot, add near-boiling water and infuse for 10 to 20 minutes, testing that the flavor is not becoming too bitter. Strain the liquid into a stoppered bottle. Add honey, grated lemon zest from one lemon and squeezed juice from both, and store in the fridge. After a day or two there will be a sediment, so filter the lemonbalmade through a coffee filter. It will keep in the fridge for several weeks.

Serving: It can be served chilled and neat, or diluted half-and-half with sparkling water. The infusion can also be used in cocktail mixes (alcoholic or nonalcoholic), or added to fruit salads or any other dish that requires lemon juice.

HOW TO TAKE IT: Our favorite for a fresh tea that can be drunk several times a day hot or cold (4 to 8 g fresh or 2 to 4 g dried per 240 ml water) or drink lemonbalmade. Harvest leaves when the sun is out and before flowering, when essential oil concentration is at its highest. Also used in many herbal liqueurs and culinary dishes including salads, soups, marinades, and dressings (trout stuffed with fresh leaves is delicious). Essential oil is used in aromatherapy and is one of the most expensive, so beware of adulterated products. Tinctures, tablets, and capsules also used.

SAFETY: Like lavender, lemon balm is one of the safest medicinal plants. Side effects are not reported and the plant (not the essential oil) is widely recommended for children. No data on contraindications, except hypothyroidism (lemon balm is used traditionally for hyperthyroid). No data for use in pregnancy. The essential oil can cause skin irritation. Lemon balm is approved by Germany's Commission E for nervous sleep disorders.

Rhodiola rosea syn. *Sedum roseum*

ROSEROOT

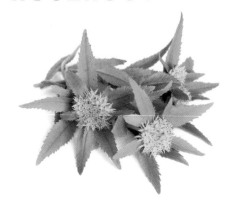

Roseroot has a widespread reputation for relieving mental fatigue and stress, enhancing physical performance and enhancing mood and memory.

ABOUT THE PLANT: This perennial is found in arctic and mountainous regions from Eurasia to Japan. Slow and low-growing with fleshy leaves, yellow flowers and long, thick, yellow-colored, red-centerd roots which have a rose-like fragrance.

HISTORY AND FOLKLORE: Also called arctic root, golden root, and Aaron's rod (implying magical powers), this plant was greatly valued by the ancient Greeks, Vikings, and Mongolians for health and vitality. Used in Siberia by shamans to help them endure all-night rituals, it is still said in Siberia that people who drink the tea will live to be a hundred. The first report of its medicinal use dates back to Greek physician Dioscorides in his *Materia Medica*. Eastern and Western medical herbalists today prescribe it for depression and as a tonic to increase performance, as an adaptogen to build strength and immune function after illness and trauma, to help cope with stress (and especially cold or high altitude), and also to improve libido in men and women, among a range of other bodily benefits.

WHAT SCIENTISTS SAY

In humans: Clinical trial evidence for roseroot consists of contradictory findings, as it does for ginseng, another adaptogen. Here we cite positive results that confirm traditional use.

For calming and blues-busting In controlled trials roseroot extracts reduced anxiety and depression in the moderately anxious and in mild to moderate depression with no serious side effects and with fewer drug interactions than for the more widely used St. John's wort. Compared with the drug sertraline, roseroot was not as effective, but had less side effects, which suggested a better benefit to risk ratio.

For memory In controlled trials, roseroot improves cognitive function in doctors on night duty, capacity for mental work in 162 cadets, and performance in mental fatigue in students. In a trial in combination with two other plants, it improved attention, speed, and accuracy in stressful cognitive tasks. In a trial that was not placebo-controlled, it improved memory in 120 adults, results being better with a higher dose.

For energy In combination with Siberian ginseng (*Eleutherococcus senticosus*) and schisandra (*Schisandra chinensis*), roseroot increased mental working capacity in healthy volunteers. In a controlled study roseroot reduced stress-related fatigue and cortisol response to stress, and increased mental performance and the ability to concentrate. In pilot trials it reduced stress-related and muscle fatigue and increased stamina in exercise, high-altitude training in athletes, burn out, and CFS. These contrast with the results of one controlled study where roseroot increased fatigue.

For sleep Roseroot improved sleep at high altitude as effectively as a hypnotic drug where REM increased and wakefulness decreased.

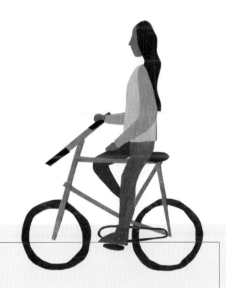

Outdoor healing

Exercise is one of the chief ways of maintaining both mental and physical health. The latest finding is that it reduces inflammatory processes that are implicated in brain cognition and mood and body reactions to stress and ill health. It raises brain growth factors that promote growth, survival, and protection of neurons and even generates new brain cells and improves mood, cognition, and sleep.

In the lab: Relieves stress and depressive behaviors with the chemicals rosavin and salidroside being specifically antidepressant. Antianxiety effects are not by the usual brain calming (GABA) signal or excitatory (glutamate), raising the possibility of new mechanisms. Extract and salidroside affect dopamine and lower release of cortisone and stress kinases (which play a role in overactivity during the stress reaction), as well as inhibit the sensitivity of signals (receptors) to cortisol—a feature in people with major depression. These effects are similar to the adaptogen ginseng. Improves memory in lab models that mimic age-related memory changes and relieves cognitive deficits in models of Alzheimer's. Reduces reward effects of cocaine and helps withdrawal from nicotine, suggesting an application in drug addiction. Also pain relieving in lab models, and improves breathing and ventilation (blood oxygen) efficiency.

KEY INGREDIENTS: Cinnamic glycosides rosin, rosavin (antidepressant), and rosarin, and phenols such as salidroside (similar in structure to catecholamines and potentially contributing to adaptogenic mechanisms). Also a volatile oil containing calming terpenes such as geraniol and citronellal.

HOW TO TAKE IT: Commonly taken as capsules of powdered root, tablets, or tinctures. Root fresh or dried also taken as a tea, although alcoholic root extracts are said to be more effective than water extracts.

SAFETY: Regarded as safe and nonaddictive though side effects such as anxiety, agitation, or insomnia, common to other mild stimulants, can occasionally occur. Higher doses may be sedative. Drug interactions are not reported, though inhibition of liver enzyme (CYP2C9) may mean caution with other drugs such as phenytoin and warfarin.

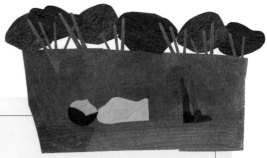

The Alexander Technique in a lavender garden

Learning the Alexander Technique can revolutionize the way in which you use your body. It teaches you to become aware of the way you move, and you will probably discover that you can do so much more naturally and easily. When you begin with the Alexander Technique you may notice that your shoulders are up near your ears or that you are not moving your hips freely. We develop all kinds of tensions as a result of a sedentary way of life, and in time with a good teacher you will become more conscious of the way you move and enjoy the benefits that come from practicing in a chosen space such as a lavender or lemon balm garden.

Panax ginseng (Chinese/Asian) and *Panax quinquefolius* (American)

GINSENG

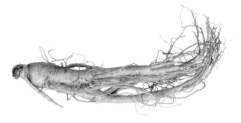

Ginseng, the world's best-selling and best-known Chinese medicinal plant for vitality, has emerging evidence (disputed by some) of benefits for mood, sleep, pain, and sex life, as well as its more established cognitive and general body benefits. The *Panax* genus may deserve its name, which has the same origin as the word "panacea." Like roseroot, there is no comparable treatment in mainstream Western medicine.

ABOUT THE PLANT: A slow-growing perennial with fleshy roots, native to the Far East, *P. ginseng* is now very rare in the wild, and should therefore be sourced from a cultivated crop. *P. quinquefolius* is a perennial growing to 39 inches (1 m), with five lobed oval leaves growing in a circle (hence its name five fingers), it's related to ivy (*Hedera* species), with small greenish-white flowers that fruit to its classic small head of clustered red berries. Its succulent, aromatic, brownish-yellow root is used medicinally after four years' growth (root hairs are not used). Siberian "ginseng" (*Eleutherococcus senticosus*), from a different genus but in the same family, is also used.

HISTORY AND FOLKLORE: Panax means all-healing in Greek, from the goddess Panacea, who healed all illness. Ginseng comes from Chinese *rénshe-n, rén* meaning person and *she-n* root (which in ginseng is suggestive of the human form). Valued for more than 6,000 years in traditional Chinese medicine, ginseng is used as a tonic to revitalize and to restore the body's *qi* (energy). Ancient Chinese emperors valued it more than gold, and wars were fought over land where it thrived. *P. quinquefolius*, used by Native Americans, was discovered by a Jesuit priest who set up trade with China.

In both the East and West ginseng is used not just as a medicine but as a stimulating tonic for young people to improve mental and physical performance and resistance to stress. Taken as a restorative tonic to improve memory and health in the elderly, it's also used in diseases such as anorexia, digestive complaints, heart failure, and depression, and also as a sedative and for mental and physical exhaustion—when the body requires sleep. The Chinese consider American ginseng milder than Asian. In China it's also an aphrodisiac.

WHAT SCIENTISTS SAY

In humans: With many clinical studies short on subject numbers, not randomized or controlled, or negative in outcome, we cite studies with positive effects. Studies relate to *P. ginseng* unless stated otherwise.

For calming Ginseng improved aspects of anxiety and increased self-reported calm in students in controlled trials. It reduces symptoms of stress during mental tasks in combination with other plants; anxiety with fibromyalgia; symptoms of attention deficit disorder in children; and symptoms of alcohol hangovers.

For blues-busting and sleep With other plants, and the drug donepezil, ginseng improves mood and behavioral measures in

Alzheimer's. It also improves quality of sleep in cancer patients and increases slow wave sleep and lowers rapid eye movement sleep in healthy males.

For memory American ginseng, with ginkgo and saffron, improved memory in controlled trials in healthy adults and also in schizophrenia, chronic fatigue syndrome (CFS), and Alzheimer's. *P. quinquefolius* also enhances memory and reduces Parkinson-like movement disorder in schizophrenia. Chinese ginseng and American ginseng may have distinct actions on memory, and there may be different dose effects. A Cochrane review on memory concluded that "analysis suggests improvement of some aspects of cognitive function, behavior and quality of life.

For energy In controlled trials, ginseng improved performance and well-being, decreased fatigue, and increased work capacity in healthy people during exercise. It relieved fatigue including aiding recovery, reduced blood markers of oxidative stress, improved pulmonary function and exercise capacity with chronic obstructive pulmonary disease, and enhanced immune responses.

For pain Controlled but not randomized studies in China show ginseng (and other closely related species) relieve pain in osteoarthritis and improve pain index in rheumatoid arthritis, and relieve muscle soreness in male athletes. Ginseng is also shown to increase sexual function, improve male fertility, and treat menstrual problems, and for stroke a Cochrane review (2008) states that notoginseng (*Panax notoginseng*) improves neurological outcome after a stroke though further studies are needed.

In the lab: A huge number of reports for *P. ginseng*—exceeding those for other all-rounder balms—show actions in models relevant

to anxiety, depression, cognition, stress resistance, and addiction. Ginsenosides are transformed by intestinal bacteria so studies on other modes of administration are cautioned.

For calming Saponins and certain ginsenosides are antianxiety, and extracts affect the brain calming signal (GABA) and relieve morphine and alcohol withdrawal, potentiate opioid analgesia, and counter effects of addictive drugs and development of tolerance to morphine (though not via opioid or GABA signals).

For blues-busting Ginseng and its polysaccharides are antidepressant, as are certain ginsenosides acting through brain signals for serotonin, noradrenaline, and dopamine.

For energy Ginseng and certain metabolites of ginsenosides affect the pituitary-adrenal response to stress, increasing resistance to a wide range of stress (mental and physical) through immune, antifatigue, and lowering fight or flight activity. These studies support the traditional adaptogen use for ginseng. The total effect of root is stimulatory, while some ginsenosides (predominant in American ginseng) are sedative in lab models.

For cognition Extracts reverse learning impairment and activate glutamate (NMDA), acetylcholine (nicotinic) and serotonin receptors. Different doses may have different effects on performance with, for example, 10 mg or 30 mg standardized ginseng extract producing different (not dose-related) responses in lab models of memory. Extracts and ginsenosides are neuroprotective through several mechanisms such as enhancing outgrowth, regenerating neuronal networks, and protecting from various types of toxicity including against one that induces Parkinsonism in models. There is a lower incidence of Parkinson's in China, where ginseng is widely consumed.

KEY INGREDIENTS: The wide variety of saponin ginsenosides are key actives, the ratio and content increasing with root age—threefold in first four years. Also contains active polysaccharides, peptides, lipids and an essential oil containing sesquiterpenes. Different species do not have the same composition but all contain saponin ginsenosides in different proportions.

HOW TO TAKE IT: Dried root is traditionally taken sliced, in Asia 1 to 10 g per day, and in the West 0.5 to 3 g per day. In Korea, ginseng-infused tea (*insamcha*) and liqueur (*insamju*) are consumed, and in China it's added to soups. Dried root is "white," but when steamed then dried, it's "red" ginseng—the steam processing is said to increase potency and it does change constituents and their ratios. Root is also chewed, and fluid extracts, tablets and capsules of powdered root are available. Recommended to take for up to three months in the West but in the East it is often used continuously in the unwell and elderly.

SAFETY: Ginseng has a good safety profile for short-term use. Side effects such as high blood pressure, headaches, insomnia, and digestive problems are sometimes reported in long-term or overuse. Caution with warfarin, monoamine oxidase inhibitors, and hypoglycemics, and in acute asthma and fever, excessive menstruation, nose bleeds, and before major surgery. Ginseng is used as a tonic in pregnancy in Asia. It's in the Chinese, Japanese, European, United States, French (since 1989), and British pharmacopoeias. Beware adulterated products such as those adulterated with the stimulant ephedrine.

Theobroma cacao

COCOA

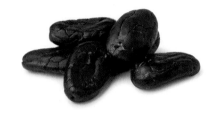

A "tree of life" for heart and mind with seed extracts that enhance mood and memory, reduce stress and pain, and are energizing and neuroprotective.

ABOUT THE PLANT: A small (26 feet/8 m) evergreen tree native to tropical regions of Central and South America, with long, broad leaves and yellowish-white or pale pink flowers said to be among the most beautiful and unusual in the world, since they grow directly out of the trunk and, being unscented, are pollinated not by bees but by midges and other jungle insects. Cocoa beans are contained in pods that vary in color from white or yellow to purple and green and are bitter until fermented or roasted.

HISTORY AND FOLKLORE: Cocoa was consumed more than 5,000 years ago by pre-Columbian cultures along the Yucatán, including the Aztecs and Mayans, who revered it as a source of divine ambrosia bestowed upon them by their great god Quetzalcoatl and used it in spiritual ceremonies. The bean was a common currency in South America before the Spanish conquest. In the sixteenth century, the Spanish chronicler Sahagún reported cocoa "especially that made with the green young fruits has the power to intoxicate, to make one dizzy and to make one drunk." He warns against drinking too much, though agrees that when taken in moderation it fortifies body and spirit. The eighteenth-century Swedish botanist Carl Linnaeus, acknowledging its reputation as a food of the gods, gave it its Latin name (*theo* for god and *broma* for food). It's used in plant medicine today to improve mood, as a diuretic, especially in heart disease, and for blood pressure control.

WHAT SCIENTISTS SAY

In humans: Studies mostly relate to consuming high-cocoa, polyphenol-enriched, low-milk content chocolate.

For calming and blues-busting Improvements in calmness and contentment, while significant, are complicated by the effects of comfort-eating sweet foods. In a pilot study dark chocolate reduced stress levels of cortisol, and in controlled trials eating chocolate reduced anxiety and depression in obese people and improved contentment in the middle-aged. High-cocoa chocolate improved mood and cognition during sustained mental effort. Higher than normal consumption of chocolate in people with Parkinson's disease and depression may reflect self-stimulation of brain amines (dopamine and serotonin effects) involved in these conditions.

For memory Most but not all controlled studies show improvement in cognition in adults, the elderly, and those with mild cognitive impairment. Brain imaging identifies increased functioning of a key memory area (the dentate gyrus in the hippocampus) and cocoa counters effects of sleep deprivation on cognition. Correlations between chocolate consumption and the chance of being a Nobel laureate are striking but not necessarily causal!

For energy Cocoa lowered fatigue in healthy adults in a controlled trial. It relieves symptoms of CFS and promotes postexercise recovery in athletes, as well as reducing blood markers of oxidative stress.

For pain Eating hedonic foods such as chocolate increases tolerance of pain. Cocoa decreased pain after exercise and increased pain tolerance in a cold environment in pilot studies.

In the lab: Methylxanthines such as theobromide enhance the effect of pleasure, pain-blocking, and attention signals such as dopamine, cannabinoid, and acetylcholine, inhibit a sleep signal (adenosine), interact with the calming (GABA) signal, improve memory models, lower inflammatory proteins, as well as affect other brain signals. Flavonoids, in addition to being antioxidant, also increase cerebral blood flow, the growth of blood vessels, and are neuroprotective, neurogenic (promote new brain neurons), and promote connectivity between neurons. Cocoa extracts, and its constituent epicatechin, promote cognition and are neuroprotective in several age- and cognitive-decline-related lab models.

KEY INGREDIENTS: Alkaloid methylxanthines (also in tea, coffee, and stimulant drinks) such as the stimulant theobromine, which is milder than caffeine and present to a lesser extent than in coffee, caffeine, and theophyllene (the bronchial dilator). Amines such as phenethylamine (a stimulant similar to amphetamine), tyramine, and histamine and cannabinoid-like fatty acid compounds (N-acylethanolamines; also in other plants such as tomatoes and peas) mimic or enhance the brain's own cannabinoid signal. A rich source of phenols such as flavonoid procyanidins and flavonols such as epicatechin (also in green tea), which is a strong antioxidant while also being insulin-like and improving heart and other health.

HOW TO TAKE IT: Ground raw cocoa beans are likely to have more health benefits than chocolate since, apart from the lack of added sugar and milk, some protective polyphenol chemicals such as cathechin are reduced by high roasting temperatures. But they're not as tasty as the processed roasted bean—a small piece (around ⅓ ounce/10 g) of dark chocolate (at least 70 percent cocoa) daily is frequently recommended.

SAFETY: Can trigger migraines and heart arrhythmias (due to amines). Drug interactions include nonsteroidal anti-inflammatories and anticoagulants. Dangerous for dogs!

Brain balm truffles

Combine the following ingredients in a food processor and pulse until they stick together. Divide the mixture into 24 small balls and roll in cocoa powder to finish. Store in the fridge for up to 5 days.

1 pound (450 g) pitted dates
1 cup (100 g) ground almonds
4 teaspoons (15 g) chia seeds
4 teaspoons (15 g) flaxseed
3 tablespoons cocoa powder
4 tablespoons agave syrup
2 tablespoons cashew milk
1 teaspoon lavender flowers
1 tablespoon lemon balm leaves
1 teaspoon powdered roseroot or ginseng

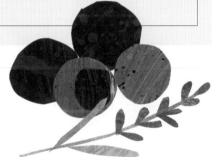

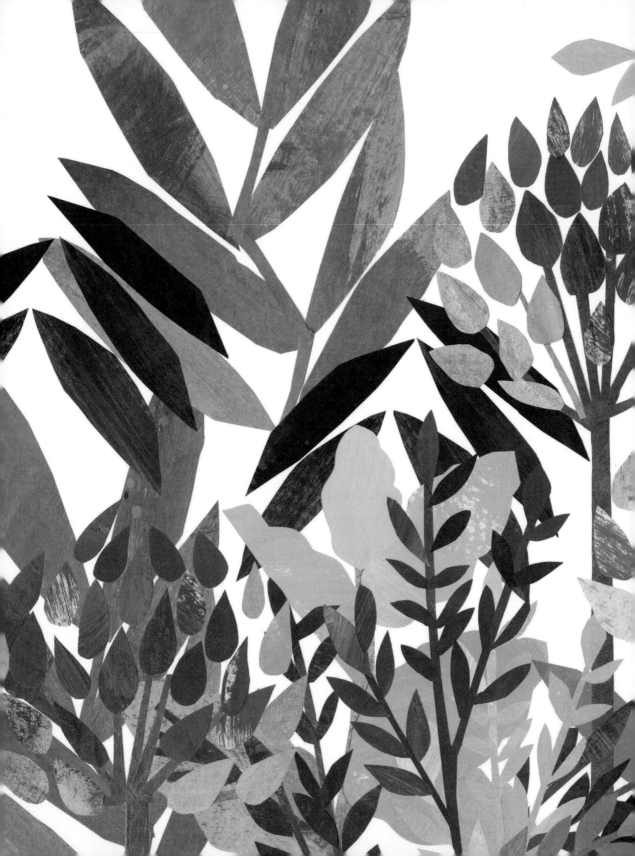

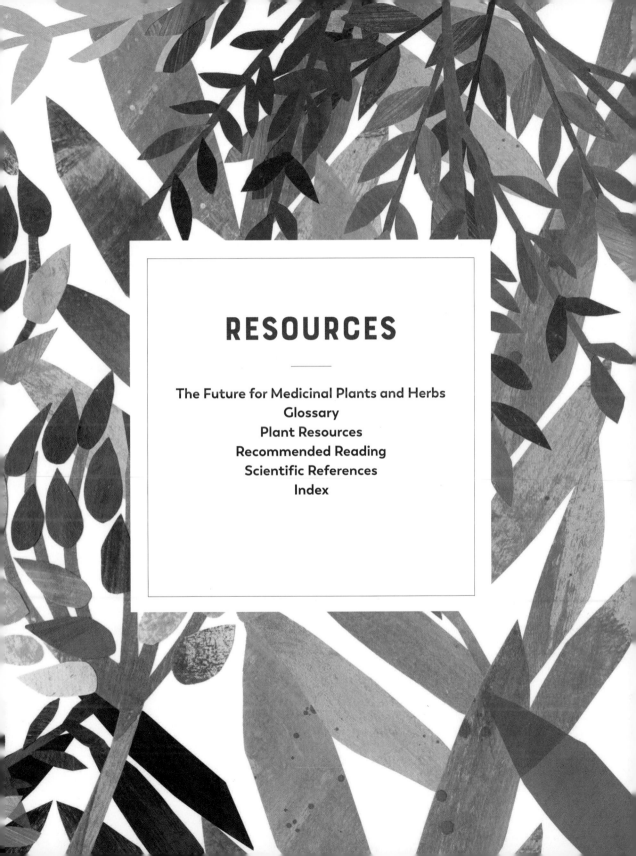

RESOURCES

The Future for Medicinal Plants and Herbs
Glossary
Plant Resources
Recommended Reading
Scientific References
Index

The Future for Medicinal Plants and Herbs

Humans have been using plants for health for over 2,000 years but it is only now that we are beginning to understand the science. Prospects for botanical brain balms are great: as whole plant "multidrugs" to take on modern drugs, as a potential source of powerful new cognitive drugs, and for their significant potential as neuroprotectants. The last three decades have seen exponential scientific research into plants for the brain, and those plants that have been sufficiently studied, for example St. John's wort for mood, arnica and cayenne for pain, kava for calming, and valerian for sleep, are standing at a new frontier in medical science. Although many more trials on brain balms and lab tests on their mechanisms are needed, this book highlights just how important the emerging clinical science on traditionally used brain balms is. As we draw to a conclusion, our thoughts look to the future of botanical brain balms and three areas stand out.

ADAPTOGENS—THE VALUE OF PLANTS FOR CHRONIC STRESS

Plants known as adaptogens are used in plant medicine to help people cope with stress and chronic disease—they are said to boost, protect, and help "adapt" or normalize body systems under chronic stress. This book contains plant adaptogens such as ginseng, bacopa, gotu kola, and roseroot that are used widely in Asia and Europe, and there are other plant adaptogens such as damiana (*Turneria diffusa*) used in South America. There is no drug equivalent

to an adaptogen, and the European Medicines Agency reported (2008) certain plants act in a number of ways (a network pharmacology) to boost resistance to stress (regulating cortisol and stimulating immunity and neuroprotection), but that clinical evidence is lacking. Clinical trials do show that adaptogens like roseroot and Siberian ginseng relieve depression, anxiety, and fatigue and increase mental capacity during stress, as well as clinically alter stress mediators.

A fascinating aspect of plant adaptogens is that they are said to normalize body systems and thus may produce different effects that depend on the biological state of the individual—in the unwell and in the healthy for example. We're all biologically and genetically individual and our bodily states are susceptible to effects from our own current environment, so we know a drug or multidrug from a plant is likely to produce different effects in different people—an aspect medical herbalists focus on in prescriptions.

EPIGENETICS—SWITCHING GENES ON AND OFF TO CHANGE YOUR MIND

The way we think, feel, and use our brains affects the body in obvious ways (heart rate, gut function, muscle tension) but also remarkably actually turns our genes on and off in the long term (epigenetics). The work of Dr. Bruce Lipton and other epigenetic researchers shows that it's not just environmental signals (like drugs, alcohol, and lack of vitamin D) but also thoughts, emotions, and stress that directly affect DNA expression in lab models. "I think therefore I am" could have yet another level of meaning. Unexpectedly some epigenetic changes may be passed down to the first and even second generation. So for chronic states of stress, anxiety, or depressed mood, any way of "normalizing" or "optimizing" brain function

> "All that man needs for health
> and healing has been provided by God
> in nature, the challenge of science is to find it."
> —Paracelsus

has to be worth considering. Plants that affect the brain may alter its gene expression, so botanical brain balms that safely help us stay calm, sleep well, think clearly, maintain a good mood, feel happy could have longer effects than you might imagine.

PLANT BREEDING—THE FUTURE FOR MEDICINAL PLANTS AND HERBS?

The possibility that plants and animals evolve together is supported by the idea that some plants adapt their chemicals to strengthen animal memory systems so that pollinating or propagating animals remember to return to that particular plant again. The same could apply in other ways—mood-lifting chemicals that engage the propagator for longer, soporific chemicals that protect against predators. But what if, for these brain balm plants, humans were to push the button to make genetic changes more in their favor by selective breeding, as we already do for certain constituents of food crops, for example omega-3 fatty acids? Could we breed a more calming lavender or more cognitive-enhancing sage? The answer has to be yes—as we've already seen cannabis bred for higher THC levels over the centuries. Perhaps this is one way forward for the pharmaceutical industry to benefit from plants as medicine. Speculation such as this can sow seeds for much needed new scientific experiment and understanding.

Glossary

ACETYLCHOLINE (ACH) is a key transmitter involved in attention and memory and it decreases as we age and in Alzheimer's Disease. It's made from choline, which is partly gained from diet, so increasing choline in the diet (soy and quinoa are choline-rich plants) may increase ACh levels.

ADAPTOGEN An herbal medicine term used for plants that protect or boost body systems that are disturbed by or involved in chronic stress or disease, for example the neuroendocrine and immune systems. An adaptogen helps the body "adapt" to stress.

ADENOSINE A chemical that builds up in the brain during the day, inducing sleep, that has other important roles such as in the cardiovascular system, pain management, and disease. Caffeine blocks the action of adenosine.

ADHD Attention Deficit Hyperactivity Disorder. A complex disorder associated with a range of behavioral manifestations and with significant impairment in functioning.

ALKALOIDS Constituents in plants that contain a nitrogen atom, for example morphine, quinine, nicotine, and caffeine. There are over 20,000 different structures.

ANTI-INFLAMMATORY A chemical or plant that can decrease inflammation, which is associated with various diseases in the brain and other parts of the body.

ANTIOXIDANT A chemical or plant that can decrease oxidation, which in excess is associated with disease.

AROMATHERAPY A practice that uses a plant's aromatic (volatile) chemicals that are present in essential oils, for improving mental well-being. Since most of the active ingredients of essential oil are small, oily, and volatile, the best methods of allowing them to reach the brain are by massage, inhalation, dermal patches, sprays, and room diffusers. *See also* Essential oil.

AYURVEDIC medicine is an ancient Indian approach to health that considers disease as "the mind and body out of health with its environment" and looks to remedy it with herbs, diets, and other therapies.

BIOACTIVE A chemical that is biologically active. A neuroactive chemical affects nerve cells. Neurotransmitters are bioactive because they result in a change in activity.

BENZODIAZEPINE A drug that acts on the brain signal receptor (also called benzodiazepine) to increase the brain's calming (GABA) neurotransmitter to produce antianxiety and sedative effects.

BRAIN mechanisms and neurochemicals in the brain (their signals, neurons, and connections) are studied through psychology (mind and behavior), neurogenetics (DNA and anatomy), neuroimaging (linking areas of the brain to function, like the hippocampus to memory or the amygdala to emotions), electrophysiology (neuron networks and electrical impulses), and neurotransmitters (*see* Acetylcholine). The difference between the brain's different signal systems is location—where the neurons are in the brain, what areas each connects with, and what neuron networks that control different brain functions they activate. Acetylcholine neurons in the base of the forebrain connect with the hippocampus and control memory. Dopamine neurons in the midbrain connect with the prefrontal cortex and govern drive and reward mechanisms. Serotonin neurons in the brainstem are linked to many cortical and other brain areas and control mood and emotion. The endogenous opioid (endorphin and encephalin) systems are distributed through the brain and spinal cord, neurons in the brainstem decreasing activity in ascending pathways for pain stimuli.

CANNABINOID The body's endogenous (inbuilt) cannabinoids such as anandamide are found in the brain as well as other parts of the body and are involved in pain and pleasure as well as immune and other functions. In cannabis, CBD (cannabidiol) is sedative, whereas THC (tetrahydrocannabinol) is mind altering.

CAPSULE A capsule contains finely chopped, ground, or powdered dried plant material sold commercially and often used in clinical trials. Take as instructed.

CFS Chronic Fatigue Syndrome or Myalgic Encephalomyelitis is an illness with a range of symptoms, long-term fatigue being the most predominant, that limit daily activities.

CLAUSTRUM is a thin structure in the center of the brain that sends information to and from many regions of the cortex and has, among other parts of the brain, been implicated in conscious awareness.

CLINICAL evidence or controlled trials include the "gold standard," which are randomized double-blind placebo-controlled trials (RCT): "placebo-controlled" where the substance is tested alongside an inert "pill" that has no effect, "blind" where no one knows who is taking test or placebo and "randomized" where people in the test and placebo groups are split up randomly.

In this book we include other pilot trial evidence from uncontrolled or open label trials. Most plant trials use under 100 participants compared to pharmaceutical drug trials which use hundreds or thousands, but as long as the difference between the test plant and placebo or between the start and end of the trial are statistically significant, the result is valid.

We cite the trials that support the traditional uses of the plant but also note if there are substantial negative outcomes.

CNS Central Nervous System comprises the brain and spinal cord in vertebrates and is responsible for controlling the activity of the mind and body; it does not include the peripheral nerves.

COCHRANE review is a systematic review that attempts to appraise all the empirical (largely clinical) evidence that meets eligible criteria, of a plant's or drug's efficacy.

COMPRESS is a pad of bruised plant material applied directly to the skin for pain and wound healing.

CORTISOL is the predominant hormone produced by the adrenal gland, involved in the stress and immune response.

DECOCTION is the extraction of the water-soluble bioactives by simmering to more forcefully extract the active ingredients from tough plant matter such as root, bark, berries, or peel. A standard daily decoction for plants used as foodstuffs is 1.41 ounces (40 g) fresh or 0.71 ounces (20 g) dried in 3 cups (750 ml) cold water, reduced to 2 cups (500 ml) after simmering.

DOPAMINE is the brain's main reward and pleasure signal that is also involved in other functions such as addiction, motivation, movement, and memory consolidation. Dopamine together with noradrenaline and serotonin is the target of some antidepressants (less used now) that block the enzyme monoamine oxidase (MAO) that breaks them down, and so increase their levels in the brain.

ENDORPHINS, the brain's own opiates, are chemicals that act on the brain's inbuilt endorphin or encephalin pain pathways via opiate receptors, and are involved in pleasure, reward, and addiction.

EPIDEMIOLOGICAL study. A study of geographical populations as they are (without intervention) to analyze disease prevalence. Some look at habits (such as food consumption) of certain populations against disease prevalence (dementia, cardiovascular disorders, or longevity, for example). They indicate but do not prove cause and effect.

ESSENTIAL oils are the highly concentrated aromatic portion of a plant and like dried plant material can contain more than one bioactive ingredient with diverse effects from antimicrobial, antioxidant and anti-inflammatory to clinically calming, stimulating or antidepressant. Always source a pure essential oil from a reputable company because oils can be adulterated with other cheaper oils or chemicals. Although some essential oils are toxic and must not be taken internally, many are given "generally recognized as safe" (GRAS) status for internal use in food products. Always use sparingly at 1 to 2 drops, diluting to 1 to 2% for daily skin application. Legally, if you make a skin product to sell or give as a gift, it must contain no more than 1% essential oil. Some essential oils can cause allergic reaction and some are phototoxic and can cause reactions when exposed to sunlight. Consult reputable aromatherapy sources for information.

FLAVONOID A group of polyphenol plant constituents responsible for the color of fruits and vegetables and commonly known for their presence in tea and wine. Although the bioavailability of some is questioned, many are health-giving. Apigenin in chamomile, quercetin in blueberries, and naringin in citrus fruits are all flavonoids.

GABA is the main calming (inhibitory) neurotransmitter in the CNS and it inhibits (or blocks) neuronal activity. Boosting its action induces feelings of calm and reduces anxiety. Benzodiazepine antianxiety drugs and a number of calming plants act to increase the efficiency of GABA (by modulating the GABAA receptor and via other mechanisms).

GLUTAMATE is the main excitatory transmitter; it stimulates (enhances) neuronal activity. It is involved in learning and memory and it is also a signal to block in order to calm and sedate. Linalool, the active ingredient in lavender and other calming plants, blocks glutamate (NMDA) receptors.

GOLD Standard trials. Controlled clinical trials on humans. *See* Clinical evidence.

GRAS US Food and Drug Administration classification of a substance that is "generally regarded as safe" by experts for consumption in foodstuffs.

HIPPOCAMPUS is part of the brain best known for its role in memory formation and consolidation. It is located in the temporal cortex and named for its shape (*hippocampus* is Greek for seahorse).

LABORATORY studies. Plants or their chemicals are tested on molecules or cells (*in vitro*) or in animal models (*in vivo*). They are significant if independent research groups show similar effects in a variety of different study types for one effect. These studies provide vital information on how, but not if, the plant works on the human brain, though changes in animal behavior indicate that they will. Trials in human subjects are the only way

to find out if the traditional use of a plant is backed up by modern medical evidence.

MELATONIN is the brain's main hormone involved in the sleep/wakefulness cycle. Increased levels induce sleep.

META-ANALYSIS is a review of several independent trials that have shown a plant's efficacy. This is the highest level of clinical evidence and several meta-analyses provide the most reliable information. It assesses the quality of trials and statistically analyzes those that are deemed methodologically sound for efficacy.

ME Myalgic Encephalomyelitis. *See* CFS.

MS Multiple sclerosis is a CNS disease that decreases myelin, a sheath on the nerve fibers that is key to fast nerve transmission, thereby disrupting electrical impulses to and from the brain.

MULTIDRUG A term used to describe the polypharmaceutical nature of plants that contain more than one bioactive chemical constituent.

NEUROPROTECTION A compound is neuroprotective if it preserves the structure and function of brain cells, for example by preventing oxidation and inflammation, actions that are also fundamental to maintaining the health of plants and the animals that consume them. Also important is countering protein deposits from cellular degeneration that occur naturally in the aging brain (and plant!) and contribute to mild cognitive impairment, Alzheimer's or Parkinson's. Promoting neurogenesis (the growth of neurones) and neuroplasticity (the formation of new neurons) underpins brain function, and studies show such effects by plant chemicals. Though studying neuroprotection clinically requires long-term trials, lab studies show many plant molecules, from polyphenols to alkaloids, are neuroprotective by different mechanisms.

NEUROTRANSMITTERS are endogenous chemicals that transmit messages between nerve cells in the brain and nerves cells and organs in the body. How molecules in the plant and molecules in the brain talk to each other (interact) is key to understanding how plants and drugs affect brain function. There are around 100 brain neurotransmitter signals that link cells together and in this book we focus on the key signals involved in different brain functions. Depending on where in the brain these signals are, their function can vary. We have given them user-friendly names like mood-boosting (serotonin/5HT and dopamine), calm (promoting the brain's inhibitory GABA or blocking the stimulatory glutamate), pain (opioid, dopamine, cannabinoid), memory and attention (acetylcholine, glutamate), sleep (adenosine, melatonin, GABA and glutamate), and pleasure or reward (cannabinoid, opioid, dopamine). One or more of these signals may be altered by drugs or a plant chemical.

NORADRENALINE, also known as norepinephrine, is a neurotransmitter and hormone involved in attention, perception, and memory and is known for "fight, flight, or freeze" responses.

OINTMENTS, along with lotions, creams, and infused oils, are topical applications made from heat-extracted plant material such as arnica or comfrey and/or essential oils, in a carrier oil, cream, or wax. Used for local application to relieve pain (e.g., arthritic, rheumatic, or from injury), increase blood flow, and speed wound healing. Also used as a means by which the oily aromatic bioactives in essential oils are absorbed into the blood and reach the brain (bypassing gut and liver metabolism).

OPIOIDS are drugs or plant chemicals that relieve pain by targeting the brain's opioid receptors, which are involved in pain and reward. Morphine in opium poppy is an opioid.

PHARMACOPOEIA is an official publication that describes drugs and potential bioactive chemicals from plants for health and medicine.

PHENOLICS, also known as phenols, are a group of ubiquitous plant constituents, including the flavonoid subgroup, that have multifunctional roles in a plant's interaction with its environment, largely protecting from stress. They are significant to humans because of their anti-inflammatory, antioxidant, anticancer, and other protective effects.

PINENE is a small, volatile compound found in some essential oils such as chamomile, sage, and pine. It has two "isomer" forms—alpha-pinene and beta-pinene. Alpha-pinene in the lab is calming (increases GABA), mood- and memory-boosting, as well as antioxidant and anti-inflammatory.

POLYPHARMACOLOGY can refer to a single chemical or drug having multiple actions but is more commonly used to describe a plant (or drug combination) when one or more of its constituent bioactive chemicals has more than one action.

POPULATION study. *See* Epidemiological study.

PSYCHOSIS is a disordered brain state that is not within the normal range of consciousness, in which perceptions differ from the norm and hallucinations and delusions are a feature.

REM Rapid Eye Movement occurs after around 90 minutes of sleep with further stages of longer duration occurring as sleep progresses. It is the most active stage of sleep in which vivid dreams occur most intensely.

SAPONINS are plant constituents that form a lather with water; they are present in foodstuffs such as cereals. They have a wide range of pharmacological effects including sedative and anti-inflammatory.

SEROTONIN is thought of as the brain's primary mood-boosting transmitter associated with feelings of contentment, and it's one of the main pathways for the action of antidepressant drugs, the selective serotonin reuptake inhibitors (SSRIs).

SSRI Selective Serotonin Reuptake Inhibitor. A chemical (or drug) that prevents serotonin being removed from the synapse, thereby increasing its presence and its mood-boosting effects.

STANDARDIZATION A plant medicine that has been prepared to ensure a more uniform product (and also confirms its identity and purity) for testing in clinical trials or for commercial production. This means the product contains a fixed amount of the known active ingredients for a specific disorder. Since chemicals in plants naturally vary, this is more reliable in a clinical trial setting. However, since the concentration and ratio of individual plant ingredients can be different in standardized extracts compared to the original whole plant extract, it does not necessarily reflect the total traditional medicinal benefit of the plant.

TABLET Plant medicines in tablet form can be more concentrated and are often extracted using other methods (such as other solvents or CO_2 extraction) and can contain other ingredients such as stabilizers, vitamins and other active plants. Take as instructed.

TEA A tea or infusion is the extraction of the plant's water-soluble bioactives. Medical herbalists recommend leaving the plant to infuse in the boiled water for 15 minutes, covered to prevent evaporation of volatile ingredients. A standard daily infusion for plants used as foodstuffs is 1 ounce (30 g) fresh (or 0.71 ounce/20 g dried) plant material per 2 cups (500 ml) boiled water daily.

TINCTURE is the extraction in alcohol of the oily and water-soluble bioactives, which more closely reflects the chemical content and ratio of the original plant material than a water extract. Tinctures are considered by many medical herbalists to be a more bioavailable due to esterification of constituent molecules. Also available commercially, they are often produced in concentrations such as 1:2 or 1:5 where 1 part (usually fresh) chopped plant material is placed in 2 or 5 parts alcohol. At home you can add the chopped plant to vodka or rum, for example, leave (agitating daily) for up to 2 weeks, strain, store in dark bottles, and take according to the recommend dose.

TRICYCLIC antidepressant. A drug or chemical that inhibits the enzyme MAO (*see* Dopamine), which in turn prevents the breakdown of the amine neurotransmitters (dopamine, serotonin, and noradrenaline) to boost mood.

TCM Traditional Chinese Medicine is an ancient herbal medicine system from China based around the concept of balanced *qi* (pronounced chi, meaning energy flow) that uses multiple plants combined with alternative medicine practices such as acupuncture.

Plant Resources

Consult

In order to effectively take a plant medicine for a condition, professional advice must be sought. Here are some associations that provide information and links to registered practitioners.

United Kingdom and Europe

Aromatherapy Council
http://aromatherapycouncil.co.uk

British Herbal Medicine Association
http://bhma.info

British Association of Traditional Tibetan Medicine
http://www.battm.org

College of Practitioners of Phytotherapy UK
http://thecpp.uk

European Herbal and Traditional Medicine Practitioners Association
http://ehtpa.eu/

"HerbMark" is a mark of quality issued to "practitioners who are members of professional associations affiliated to the European Herbal and Traditional Medicine Practitioners Association (EHTPA)." These professional associations are:

European Scientific Cooperative of Phytotherapy
http://escop.com

Herbalist
http://www.herbalist.org.uk

National Institute of Medical Herbalists UK
http://www.nimh.org.uk

Register of Chinese Herbal Medicine
http://rchm.co.uk

Unified Register of Herbal Practitioners
https://www.urhp.com

North America
American Botanical Council
http://abc.herbalgram.org/site/PageServer

American Herbalists Guild
https://www.americanherbalistsguild.com

The Aromatherapy Registration Council
maintains a public database of Registered
Aromatherapists and is an impartial and unbiased
body
http://www.aromatherapycouncil.org

Canadian Herbalist Association of BC
http://www.chaofbc.ca

Herb Research Foundation
http://www.herbs.org/herbnews/

Herb Society of America
http://www.herbsociety.org/

National Center for Homeopathy
http://www.homeopathycenter.org/

Rocky Mountain Herbal Institute
http://www.rmhiherbal.org/

Rest of the World

National Herbalists Association of Australia
http://www.nhaa.org.au

New Zealand Association of Medical Herbalists
http://nzamh.org.nz

HerbNET
Provides contacts for herbal associations
throughout the world although not necessarily
endorsed.
http://www.herbnet.com

Grow

United Kingdom and Europe

The Royal Horticultural Society is a valuable
resource for information on plants.
https://www.rhs.org.uk

Dilston Physic Garden was converted from
pastureland in Northumberland into the uniquely
peaceful place it is today by Elaine and Nicolette
Perry. At this modern physic garden, the Perrys
are dedicated to raising awareness of scientific
research into medicinal plants, how they can take
care of your health, and how to grow them. Visitors
may wander the pathways to discover over 800
medicinal plants with a focus on those for the
brain.
    Regular gardening activity has a positive effect
on both mind and body. A healthy body affects
the brain (circulation, metabolism, immunity for
example) and keeps it in working order. So there's
every reason to start discovering medicinal plants
and growing them for all-round health.
    Workshops and events at Dilston Physic
Garden explore a range of topics including
those below. For the latest information, go to
dilstonphysicgarden.com.

- the history of physic gardens past and present
- the science of medicinal plants including plant
  chemistry, clinical testing, comparing the
  scientific and medical herbal approaches for
  health
- choosing safe plants to grow and use for health
  and medicine that are drawn from traditional
  medical herbalism and scientific evidence
- garden design and plant cultivation
- plant formulations and ways to use plants
  for a range of purposes including first aid
  and common conditions, children's health,
  nutraceuticals, herbal teas, aromatherapy,
  cosmeceuticals, animal health, house hygiene,
  and incense

North America

Herb Society of America. Lots of information on
growing and using herbs.
http://www.herbsociety.org

North Carolina University horticultural science
http://content.ces.ncsu.edu/growing-herbs-for-the-home-gardener

Buy

Sourcing commercial plant products

The best way to check if a commercial company is reputable is through your local registered medical herbalist, pharmacist, or other professional registered practitioner who can advise where to buy plants, dried plant material, and plant medicine products in your area. Otherwise, always check that only pure plant (with the correct scientific name) is specified on the ingredients and assess the reputation of the company by descriptions, where they source their plant material, and product reviews. Quality is harder to assess for products including powdered products (as opposed to dried plant material). If they genuinely are standardized to certain chemicals (as for ginkgo and St. John's Wort) it's a sign the company is reputable. Adulteration (substituting the real plant with a cheaper plant or chemical) is not uncommon and difficult to assess if you buy powdered plant material. For example, skullcap extracts have been adulterated with germander (*Teucrium*), which causes liver toxicity.

United Kingdom

Visit the British Herbal Medicine Association (see above) for more information on products and to see a list of products (by condition) that have been given a THR (Traditional Herbal Registration) by the Medicines and Healthcare Regulatory Agency. These regulated products are widely available in health food stores and have THR stamped on their packaging.

Most of the following do mail order and smaller quantities and most have organic herbs available too:

Amphora Aromatics Ltd
https://www.amphora-retail.com

Aromantic Natural Skin Care
https://www.aromantic.co.uk

A.Vogel
https://www.avogel.co.uk

British Flora
http://www.britishflora.co.uk

G Baldwin & Co
https://www.baldwins.co.uk

Just Ingredients
https://www.justingredients.co.uk

Neals Yard Remedies
http://www.nealsyardremedies.com

Poyntzfield Herb Nursery
http://www.poyntzfieldherbs.co.uk

Seahorseandsage
http://www.seahorseandsage.com

Statfold Seed Oils (carrier oils and essential oils)
http://www.statfold-oils.co.uk

Woodland Herbs
http://www.woodlandherbs.co.uk

North America

Banyan Botanicals
www.banyanbotanicals.com

Crimson Sage Medicinal Plant Nursery
https://www.crimson-sage.com

MediHerb
http://www.standardprocess.com/MediHerb

Mountain Rose Herbs
www.mountainroseherbs.com

Find out about any adulterants by subscribing to the American Botanical Council newsletters and from adulterated herbal medicines information at http://theconversation.com/herbal-medicines-adulterated-contaminated-or-just-plain-missing-its-an-international-scandal-6060

Recommended Reading

We recommend just a few of many sources relevant to topics in the book with a particular focus on those relating to understanding the human brain and how plants and chemicals improve brain function. We also recommend sources for the identification, cultivation and use of plants as herbal medicines.

Brain & Mind

Ashton, Heather: *Brain Systems, Disorders and Psychotropic Drugs* (1992): "Brain function and psychotropic drugs." Oxford: Oxford University Press (Oxford Medical Publications).

Carter, Rita (2009): *The Brain Book*. London: Dorling Kindersley.

Collerton, Daniel; Mosimann, Urs P.; Perry, E. K. (2015): *The Neuroscience of Visual Hallucinations*. Chichester: Wiley-Blackwell.

Eagleman, David (2015): *The Brain: The Story of You*. Edinburgh: Canongate Books.

Gregory, R. L. (2004): *Oxford Companion to the Mind*. 2nd ed. Oxford: Oxford University Press.

Perry, E. K.; Collerton, Daniel; LeBeau, Fiona E. N.; Ashton, Heather (2010): *New Horizons in the Neuroscience of Consciousness*. Amsterdam, Philadelphia: John Benjamins Publishing Company (Advances in consciousness research, v. 79).

Seth, Anil K. (editor) (2014): *30-Second Brain: The 50 Most Mind-Blowing Ideas in Neuroscience, Each Explained in Half a Minute*. Foreword by Chris Frith; contributors, Tristan Bekinschtein, et al. London: Icon Books.

Webster, R. A. (2001 [2002 printing]): *Neurotransmitters, Drugs and Brain Function*. Chichester: Wiley.

Plants and the brain

Kennedy, David O. (2014): *Plants and the Human Brain*. Oxford: Oxford University Press.

Schultes, Richard Evans; Hofmann, Albert; Rätsch, Christian (2001): *Plants of the Gods: Their Sacred, Healing, and Hallucinogenic Powers*. Revised and expanded edition. Rochester, Vt.: Healing Arts Press. Available online at http://www.loc.gov/catdir/enhancements/fy0644/2001004425-b.html.

Spinella, Marcello (2001): *The Psychopharmacology of Herbal Medicine: Plant Drugs That Alter Mind, Brain, and Behavior*. Cambridge, Mass.; London: MIT Press.

Science of plant medicine

Allaby, Michael (2017): *Plant Love: The Scandalous Truth about the Sex Life of Plants*: Filbert Press.

Bruneton, Jean (1999): *Pharmacognosy, Phytochemistry, Medicinal Plants*. 2nd ed. Andover: Intercept Ltd.

Buchbauer, G.; et al. "Aromatherapy: evidence for sedative effects of the essential oil of lavender after inhalation." https://www.ncbi.nlm.nih.gov/pubmed/1817516. One of the first scientific studies showing the biological effects of inhalation of essential oils.

Cochrane Collaboration. http://www.cochrane.org/cochrane-reviews. Good source of information on efficacy and safety of medicinal plants and drugs based on meta-analysis.

Chemical Database Traditional Chinese Medicine. http://www.chemtcm.com/ Database of individual molecules, constituents of plants used in traditional Chinese herbal medicine developed at King's College London.

European Medicines Agency. http://www.ema.europa.eu/ema/index.jsp?curl=pages/home/Home_Page.jsp&mid. Agency responsible for scientific evaluation of medicines developed by pharmaceutical companies for use in European Union that provides summaries of traditional plant medicinal use including scientific research.

Natural Medicine Comprehensive Database. http://naturaldatabase.therapeuticresearch .com. Subscription reference for clinicians with "unbiased, reliable dietary supplement information" recommended by *JAMA* and the *American Journal of Medicine*.

Pengelly, A. (2004) *The Constituents of Medicinal Plants: An Introduction to the Chemistry and Therapeutics of Herbal Medicine* [2nd ed.]. Wallingford: CABI Publishing. An easy-ish introduction to plant constituents and their actions, by a medical herbalist.

Pubmed. http://www.ncbi.nlm.nih.gov/pubmed. Search engine to find scientific peer reviewed research on a medicinal plant. Comprises more than 28 million citations for biomedical literature from MEDLINE, life science journals & online books. Read the "Quick Start Guide" first: http://www.ncbi.nlm.nih.gov/books /NBK3827/#pubmedhelp.

Schulz, Volker (2011): *Rational Phytotherapy: A Physicians' Guide to Herbal Medicine*. 5th ed. Berlin, London: Springer.

WHO Monographs. http://apps.who.int /medicinedocs/en/d/Js2200e/. Series of volumes providing scientific information on the safety, efficacy, and quality control of widely used medicinal plants. Type your plant's Latin name and "WHO monograph" into your browser.

Wichtl, Max (Ed.) (2004): *Herbal Drugs and Phytopharmaceuticals: A Handbook for Practice on a Scientific Basis*. With assistance of Franz-Christian Czygan, Dietrich Frohne, Karl Hiller, Christoph Höltzel, Astrid Nagell, Peter Pachaly et al. 3 ed. Boca Raton, Fla: CRC Press.

Herbal Medicine

Bartrams, T. (1998) *The Encyclopaedia of Herbal Medicine*. London: Robinson

Blumenthal, Mark; Busse, Werner R. (1998): *The Complete German Commission E Monographs Therapeutic Guide to Herbal Medicines*. Developed by a special expert committee of the German Federal Institute for Drugs and Medical Devices. Senior editor: Mark Blumenthal; associate editors: Werner R. Busse … [et al.]; primary translator: Sigrid Klein. Austin, Tex.: American Botanical Council. The German monographs published in 1978 on the safety and efficacy of 300 plants.

Bone, Kerry; Mills, Simon (2013): *Principles and Practice of Phytotherapy: Modern Herbal Medicine*. Forewords by Michael Dixon, Mark Blumenthal. 2nd ed. Edinburgh: Churchill Livingstone.

Braun, Lesley; Cohen, Marc (2017): *Essential Herbs & Natural Supplements*. [First edition.]. Chatswood, N.S.W.: Elsevier Australia.

Chevallier, Andrew (2016): *The Encyclopedia of Herbal Medicine: 550 Herbs and Remedies for Common Ailments*. 2016, 3rd edition. New York: DK Publishing, Inc.

Chevallier, Andrew (1998): *Phytotherapy: 50 Vital Herbs*. 1st ed. Guildford, England: Amberwood Publishing.

Davis, Patricia; Budd, Sarah (2005): *Aromatherapy: An A-Z*. Revised and enlarged edition illustrated by Sarah Budd. London: Vermilion.

Duke, James A. (2002): *Handbook of Medicinal Herbs*. 2nd ed. Boca Raton, FL: CRC Press.

European Scientific Cooperative on Phytotherapy. http://escop.com/ provides authoritative profiles (monographs) on plants used as medicines—"an umbrella organisation representing national herbal medicine or phytotherapy societies across Europe . . . produces reviews of the therapeutic use of leading herbal medicinal products or herbal drug preparations based on scientific evidence and on leading expertise across Europe."

Hoffmann, David (2003): *Medical Herbalism: The Science and Practice of Herbal Medicine*. Rochester, Vt.: Healing Arts Press.

Herbalgram. http://abc.herbalgram.org/site /PageServer. *The Journal of the American Botanical Council,* containing plant-specific data and commentaries on clinical trials and adulteration.

The Herb Society UK. http://www.herbsociety.org .uk/ "promoting the use and enjoyment of herbs."

Medicine Hunter. http://www.medicinehunter .com/holy-basil. Interesting, well-written factual articles on key and unusual medicinal plants.

Mills, Simon J.; Bone, Kerry (2005): *The Essential Guide to Herbal Safety*. Edinburgh: Elsevier Churchill Livingstone.

Perry, E., and Court, D. (2014). *Tales from a Psychic Garden: In Pursuit of Herbal Happiness* (Herb Spirits Series, Book 1) Kindle Edition.

Perry, E. (2015) *Tales from a Physic Garden: Stress Less with Herbal Chill-Pills* (Herb Spirits Series, Book 2) Kindle Edition.

Perry, E., and Court, D. (2015) *Tales from a Psychic Garden: The Quest for Botanical Mood Boosters* (Herb Spirits Series, Book 3) Kindle Edition.

Tisserand, Robert; Young, Rodney (2014): *Essential Oil Safety: A Guide for Health Care Professionals*. Second edition. Edinburgh: Churchill Livingstone.

University of Maryland Medical Center lists the most commonly used herbal meds in the U.S. and their uses, doses, and precautions, and contains excellent general information on herbal medicine. https://umm.edu/health/medical/altmed /treatment/herbal-medicine.

Weiss, Rudolph Fritz (2001): *Weiss's Herbal Medicine*. Classic ed. Stuttgart: Thieme.

Herbal Medicine, Historical Use

Culpeper, N. (2007): *Culpeper's Complete Herbal*. New ed. Wordsworth Editions.

Dioscorides. *De Materia Medica*. Original herbal texts and the history of medicine, not for current medicinal use. http://www.cancerlynx. com/dioscorides.html.

Gerard, J. (1985): *Gerard's Herbal: The History of Plants*. Marcus Woodward (Editor). Bracken Books. Information on Gerard's original text. http://exhibits.hsl.virginia.edu/ herbs/herball/

Goodyer, J. (1655): *Greek Herbal of Dioscorides*. Edited by R.T. Gunter (1933).

Wren, R. C.; Williamson, Elizabeth M.; Evans, Fred J. (1988): *Potter's New Cyclopaedia of Botanical Drugs and Preparations*. Completely rev. ed. Ashingdon: C. W. Daniel Co Ltd.

Plant Identification

Barker, J. (2001): *The Medicinal Flora of Britain and NW Europe*. Winter Press.

Grey-Wilson, C. (1997): *Wild Flowers of Britain & NW Europe*. Dorling Kindersley.

Sutton, David (1993): *A Field Guide to the Wild Flowers of Britain and Northern Europe*. Parragon Plus.

Upton, Roy (2011): *American Herbal Pharmacopoeia: Botanical Pharmacognosy— Microscopic Characterization of Botanical Medicines*. Edited by: Roy Upton; et al. Boca Raton, Fl.: American Herbal Pharmacopoeia/CRC Press.

Plant Cultivation

Bonar, A. (1985). *Herbs: A Complete Guide to Their Cultivation & Use*. Hamlyn.

Green, J. (2000): *The Herbal Medicine Makers Handbook*. The Crossing Press.

Hickey, M. and King, C. (1997): *Common Families of Flowering Plants*. Cambridge University Press.

Houdret, J. (1999): *Growing Herbs*. Anness Publishing.

McIntyre, A. (1997): *The Apothecary's Garden: How to Grow and Use Your Own Herbal Medicines*. Piatkus Books.

McVicar, J. (2010): *Grow Herbs*. Dorling Kindersley.

Sinclair Rohde, E. (1936): *Herbs & Herb Gardening*. The Medici Society.

Segall, B. (1994): *The Herb Garden Month*. David & Charles.

Scientific References

We cite only scientific peer-reviewed reports for each plant. Invaluable libraries of such papers include PubMed and the Cochrane Reviews.

Care should be taken when looking at raw data in scientific articles—effects in the lab do not necessarily mean the same effects will be seen in humans; human data requires clinical data on safety and efficacy.

Introduction

van de Rest, Ondine; Am Berendsen, Agnes; Haveman-Nies, Annemien; Groot, Lisette Cpgm de (2015): "Dietary patterns, cognitive decline, and dementia: a systematic review." In *Advances in Nutrition* (Bethesda, Md.) 6 (2), pp. 154–68. DOI: 10.3945/an.114.007617.

Ng, Tze-Pin; Chiam, Peak-Chiang; Lee, Theresa; Chua, Hong-Choon; Lim, Leslie; Kua, Ee-Heok (2006): "Curry consumption and cognitive function in the elderly." In *American Journal of Epidemiology* 164 (9), pp. 898–906. DOI: 10.1093/aje/kwj267.

Hardman, Roy J.; Kennedy, Greg; Macpherson, Helen; Scholey, Andrew B.; Pipingas, Andrew (2015): "A randomised controlled trial investigating the effects of Mediterranean diet and aerobic exercise on cognition in cognitively healthy older people living independently within aged care facilities: the Lifestyle Intervention in Independent Living Aged Care (LIILAC) study protocol ACTRN12614001133628." In *Nutrition Journal* 14, p. 53. DOI: 10.1186/s12937-015-0042-z.

Dai, Qi; Borenstein, Amy R.; Wu, Yougui; Jackson, James C.; Larson, Eric B. (2006): "Fruit and vegetable juices and Alzheimer's disease: the Kame Project" In *The American Journal of Medicine* 119 (9), pp. 751–59. DOI: 10.1016/j.amjmed.2006.03.045.

Shoba, G.; Joy, D.; Joseph, T.; Majeed, M.; Rajendran, R.; Srinivas, P. S. (1998): "Influence of piperine on the pharmacokinetics of curcumin in animals and human volunteers." In *Planta medica* 64 (4), pp. 353–56. DOI: 10.1055/s-2006-957450.

Multidrug plants

Sansone, Roberto; Ottaviani, Javier I.; Rodriguez-Mateos, Ana; Heinen, Yvonne; Noske, Dorina; Spencer, Jeremy P. et al. (2017): "Methylxanthines enhance the effects of cocoa flavanols on cardiovascular function: randomized, double-masked controlled studies." In *The American Journal of Clinical Nutrition* 105 (2), pp. 352–60. DOI: 10.3945/ajcn.116.140046.

Chapter 1

Kava-Kava

Boerner, R. J.; Sommer, H.; Berger, W.; Kuhn, U.; Schmidt, U.; Mannel, M. (2003): "Kava-kava extract LI 150 is as effective as opipramol and buspirone in generalised anxiety disorder—an 8-week randomized, double-blind multi-center clinical trial in 129 out-patients." In *Phytomedicine* 10 Suppl. 4, pp. 38–49.

Malsch, U.; Kieser, M. (2001): "Efficacy of kava-kava in the treatment of non-psychotic anxiety, following pretreatment with benzodiazepines." In *Psychopharmacology* 157 (3), pp. 277–83. DOI: 10.1007/s002130100792.

Teschke, Rolf (2010): "Kava hepatotoxicity—a clinical review." In *Annals of Hepatology* 9 (3), pp. 251–65.

Ashwagandha

Jahanbakhsh, Seyedeh Pardis; Manteghi, Ali Akhondpour; Emami, Seyed Ahmad; Mahyari, Saman; Gholampour, Beheshteh; Mohammadpour, Amir Hooshang; Sahebkar, Amirhossein (2016): "Evaluation of the efficacy of *Withania somnifera* (Ashwagandha) root extract in patients with obsessive-compulsive disorder: A randomized double-blind placebo-controlled trial." In *Complementary Therapies in Medicine* 27, pp. 25–29. DOI: 10.1016/j.ctim.2016.03.018.

Pratte, Morgan A.; Nanavati, Kaushal B.; Young, Virginia; Morley, Christopher P. (2014): "An alternative treatment for anxiety: a systematic review of human trial results reported for the Ayurvedic herb ashwagandha (*Withania somnifera*)." In *Journal of Alternative and Complementary Medicine* (*New York, N.Y.*) 20 (12), pp. 901–8. DOI: 10.1089/acm.2014.0177.

Gotu Kola

Bradwejn, J.; Zhou, Y.; Koszycki, D.; Shlik, J. (2000): "A double-blind, placebo-controlled study on the effects of gotu kola (*Centella asiatica*) on acoustic startle response in healthy subjects." In *Journal of Clinical Psychopharmacology* 20 (6), pp. 680–84.

Jana, U.; Sur, T.K.; Maity, L.N.; Debnath, P.K.; Bhattacharyya, D. (2010): "A clinical study on the management of generalized anxiety disorder with *Centella asiatica*." In *Nepal Medical College Journal: NMCJ* 12 (1), pp.8–11.

Passionflower

Akhondzadeh, S.; Naghavi, H.R.; Vazirian, M.; Shayeganpour, A.; Rashidi, H.; Khani, M. (2001):

"Passionflower in the treatment of generalized anxiety: a pilot double-blind randomized controlled trial with oxazepam." In *Journal of Clinical Pharmacy and Therapeutics* 26 (5), pp. 363–67.

Aslanargun, Pınar; Cuvas, Ozgun; Dikmen, Bayazit; Aslan, Eymen; Yuksel, Mustafa Ugur (2012): "*Passiflora incarnata* Linneaus as an anxiolytic before spinal anesthesia." In *Journal of Anesthesia* 26 (1), pp. 39–44. DOI: 10.1007/s00540-011-1265-6.

Bitter Orange

Namazi, Masoumeh; Amir Ali Akbari, Seddigheh; Mojab, Faraz; Talebi, Atefe; Alavi Majd, Hamid; Jannesari, Sharareh (2014): "Aromatherapy with Citrus aurantium oil and anxiety during the first stage of labor." In *Iranian Red Crescent Medical Journal* 16 (6), e18371. DOI: 10.5812/ircmj.18371.

Pimenta, Flávia Cristina Fernandes; Alves, Mateus Feitosa; Pimenta, Martina Bragante Fernandes; Melo, Silvia Adelaide Linhares; de Almeida, Anna Alice Figueirêdo; Leite, José Roberto et al. (2016): "Anxiolytic effect of *Citrus aurantium* L. on patients with chronic myeloid leukemia." In *Phytotherapy Research*: PTR 30 (4), pp. 613–17. DOI: 10.1002/ptr.5566.

Bergamot

Hongratanaworakit, Tapanee (2011): "Aroma-therapeutic effects of massage blended essential oils on humans." In *Natural Product Communications* 6 (8), pp. 1199–1204.

Hwang, Jin-Hee (2006): "The effects of the inhalation method using essential oils on blood pressure and stress responses of clients with essential hypertension." In *Taehan Kanho Hakhoe Chi* 36 (7), pp. 1123–34.

Motherwort

Shikov, Alexander N.; Pozharitskaya, Olga N.; Makarov, Valery G.; Demchenko, Dmitry V.; Shikh, Evgenia V. (2011): "Effect of *Leonurus cardiaca* oil extract in patients with arterial hypertension accompanied by anxiety and sleep disorders." In

Phytotherapy Research : PTR 25 (4), pp. 540–43. DOI: 10.1002/ptr.3292.

Wojtyniak, Katarzyna; Szymański, Marcin; Matławska, Irena (2013): *"Leonurus cardiaca* L. (motherwort): a review of its phytochemistry and pharmacology." In *Phytotherapy Research* : PTR 27 (8), pp. 1115–20. DOI: 10.1002/ptr.4850.

Chapter 2

Don't forget your fruit and veg

Feeney, Joanne; O'Leary, Neil; Moran, Rachel; O'Halloran, Aisling M.; Nolan, John M.; Beatty, Stephen et al. (2017): "Plasma lutein and zeaxanthin are associated with better cognitive function across multiple domains in a large population-based sample of older adults: Findings from the Irish Longitudinal Study on Aging." In *The Journals of Gerontology. Series A, Biological Sciences and Medical Sciences*. DOI: 10.1093/gerona/glw330.

Vauzour, David (2014): "Effect of flavonoids on learning, memory and neurocognitive performance: relevance and potential implications for Alzheimer's disease pathophysiology." In *Journal of the Science of Food and Agriculture* 94 (6), pp. 1042–56. DOI: 10.1002/jsfa.6473.

Kean, Rebecca J.; Lamport, Daniel J.; Dodd, Georgina F.; Freeman, Jayne E.; Williams, Claire M.; Ellis, Judi A. et al. (2015): "Chronic consumption of flavanone-rich orange juice is associated with cognitive benefits: an 8-wk, randomized, double-blind, placebo-controlled trial in healthy older adults." In *The American Journal of Clinical Nutrition* 101 (3), pp. 506–14. DOI: 10.3945/ajcn.114.088518.

Chinese Clubmoss

Sun, Q.Q.; Xu, S.S.; Pan, J.L.; Guo, H.M.; Cao, W.Q. (1999): "Huperzine-A capsules enhance memory and learning performance in 34 pairs of matched adolescent students." In *Zhongguo Yao Li Xue Bao = Acta Pharmacologica Sinica* 20 (7), pp. 601–3.

Xing, Shu-Huai; Zhu, Chun-Xiao; Zhang, Rui; An, Li (2014): "Huperzine-A in the treatment of Alzheimer's disease and vascular dementia: a meta-analysis." In *Evidence-based Complementary and Alternative Medicine*: eCAM 2014, p. 363985. DOI: 10.1155/2014/363985.

Bacopa

Downey, Luke A.; Kean, James; Nemeh, Fiona; Lau, Angela; Poll, Alex; Gregory, Rebecca et al. (2013): "An acute, double-blind, placebo-controlled crossover study of 320 mg and 640 mg doses of a special extract of *Bacopa monnieri* (CDRI 08) on sustained cognitive performance." In *Phytotherapy Research*: PTR 27 (9), pp. 1407–13. DOI: 10.1002/ptr.4864.

Kongkeaw, Chuenjid; Dilokthornsakul, Piyameth; Thanarangsarit, Phurit; Limpeanchob, Nanteetip; Norman Scholfield, C. (2014): "Meta-analysis of randomized controlled trials on cognitive effects of *Bacopa monnieri* extract." In *Journal of Ethnopharmacology* 151 (1), pp. 528–35. DOI: 10.1016/j.jep.2013.11.008.

Roodenrys, Steven; Booth, Dianne; Bulzomi, Sonia; Phipps, Andrew; Micallef, Caroline; Smoker, Jaclyn (2002): "Chronic effects of Brahmi (*Bacopa monnieri*) on human memory." In *Neuropsychopharmacology* 27 (2), pp. 279–81. DOI: 10.1016/S0893-133X(01)00419-5.

Sage

Lopresti, Adrian L. (2017): "Salvia (Sage): A Review of its Potential Cognitive-Enhancing and Protective Effects." In *Drugs in R&D* 17 (1), pp. 53–64. DOI: 10.1007/s40268-016-0157-5.

Akhondzadeh, S.; Noroozian, M.; Mohammadi, M.; Ohadinia, S.; Jamshidi, A. H.; Khani, M. (2003): "Salvia officinalis extract in the treatment of patients with mild to moderate Alzheimer's disease: a double blind, randomized and placebo-controlled trial." In *Journal of Clinical Pharmacy and Therapeutics* 28 (1), pp. 53–59.

Scholey, Andrew B.; Tildesley, Nicola T. J.; Ballard, Clive G.; Wesnes, Keith A.; Tasker, Andrea; Perry, Elaine K.; Kennedy, David O. (2008):"An extract of Salvia (sage) with anticholinesterase properties improves memory and attention in healthy older volunteers." In *Psychopharmacology* 198 (1), pp. 127–39. DOI: 10.1007/s00213-008-1101-3.

Perry, N. S.; Houghton, P. J.; Sampson, J.; Theobald, A. E.; Hart, S.; Lis-Balchin, M. et al. (2001): "In-vitro activity of *S. lavandulaefolia* (Spanish sage) relevant to treatment of Alzheimer's disease." In *The Journal of Pharmacy and Pharmacology* 53 (10), pp. 1347–56.

Perry, N.S.L.; Menzies, R.; Hodgson, F.; Wedgewood, P.; Howes, M.J.R.; Brooker, H.J.; Wesnes K.A.; Perry, E.K.: "A randomised double-blind placebo-controlled pilot trial of a combined extract of sage, rosemary and melissa, traditional herbal medicines, on the enhancement of memory in normal healthy subjects, including influence of age." DOI: 10.1016/j.phymed.2017.08.015.

Nigella

Bin Sayeed, Muhammad Shahdaat; Shams, Tahiatul; Fahim Hossain, Sarder; Rahman, Md Rezowanur; Mostofa, Agm; Fahim Kadir, Mohammad et al. (2014): "*Nigella sativa* L. seeds modulate mood, anxiety and cognition in healthy adolescent males." In *Journal of Ethnopharmacology* 152 (1), pp. 156–62. DOI: 10.1016/j.jep.2013.12.050.

Javidi, Soheila; Razavi, Bibi Marjan; Hosseinzadeh, Hossein (2016): "A review of neuropharmacology effects of *Nigella sativa* and its main component, thymoquinone." In *Phytotherapy Research: PTR* 30 (8), pp. 1219–29. DOI: 10.1002/ptr.5634.

Rosemary

Moss, Mark; Cook, Jenny; Wesnes, Keith; Duckett, Paul (2003): "Aromas of rosemary and lavender essential oils differentially affect cognition and mood in healthy adults." In *The International Journal of Neuroscience* 113 (1), pp. 15–38.

Pengelly, Andrew; Snow, James; Mills, Simon Y.; Scholey, Andrew; Wesnes, Keith; Butler, Leah Reeves (2012): "Short-term study on the effects of rosemary on cognitive function in an elderly population." In *Journal of Medicinal Food* 15 (1), pp. 10–17. DOI: 10.1089/jmf.2011.0005.

Black Walnut

Arab, L.; Ang, A. (2015): "A cross-sectional study of the association between walnut consumption and cognitive function among adult US populations represented in NHANES." In *The Journal of Nutrition, Health & Aging* 19 (3), pp. 284–90. DOI: 10.1007/s12603-014-0569-2.

Blueberry

Whyte, Adrian R.; Schafer, Graham; Williams, Claire M. (2016): "Cognitive effects following acute wild blueberry supplementation in 7- to 10-year-old children." In *European Journal of Nutrition* 55 (6), pp. 2151–62. DOI: 10.1007/s00394-015-1029-4.

Take a green break at work

Taylor, Andrea Faber; Kuo, Frances E. (2009): "Children with attention deficits concentrate better after walk in the park." In *Journal of Attention Disorders* 12 (5), pp. 402–9. DOI: 10.1177/1087054708323000.

Lanki, Timo; Siponen, Taina; Ojala, Ann; Korpela, Kalevi; Pennanen, Arto; Tiittanen, Pekka et al. (2017): "Acute effects of visits to urban green environments on cardiovascular physiology in women: A field experiment." In *Environmental Research* 159, pp. 176–85. DOI: 10.1016/j.envres.2017.07.039.

Chapter 3

Ayahuasca

Dos Santos, Rafael G.; Osório, Flávia L.; Crippa, José Alexandre S.; Hallak, Jaime E. C. (2016): "Antidepressive and anxiolytic effects of ayahuasca: a systematic literature review of animal and human studies." *In Revista Brasileira de Psiquiatria* (Sao Paulo, Brazil : 1999) 38 (1), pp. 65–72. DOI: 10.1590/1516-4446-2015-1701.

St. John's Wort

Brattström, Axel (2009): "Long-term effects of St John's wort (*Hypericum perforatum*) treatment: a 1-year safety study in mild to moderate depression." In *Phytomedicine* 2009 Apr; 16 (4), pp. 277–83. DOI: 10.1016/j.phymed.2008.12.023.

Linde, K.; Ramirez, G.; Mulrow, C. D.; Pauls, A.; Weidenhammer, W.; Melchart, D. (1996): "St John's wort for depression—an overview and meta-analysis of randomised clinical trials." In *BMJ (Clinical Research Ed.)* 313 (7052), pp. 253–58.

Ng, Qin Xiang; Venkatanarayanan, Nandini; Ho, Collin Yih Xian (2017): "Clinical use of *Hypericum perforatum* (St John's wort) in depression: a meta-analysis." In *Journal of Affective Disorders* 210, pp. 211–21. DOI: 10.1016/j.jad.2016.12.048.

Turmeric

Al-Karawi, Dalia; Al Mamoori, Doaa Alem; Tayyar, Yaman (2016): "The role of curcumin administration in patients with major depressive disorder: mini meta-analysis of clinical trials." In *Phytotherapy Research : PTR* 30 (2), pp. 175–83. DOI: 10.1002/ptr.5524.

Cox, K.H., Pipingas, A., & Scholey, A.B. (2015): "Investigation of the effects of solid lipid curcumin on cognition and mood in a healthy older population." In *Journal of Psychopharmacology* 29 (5), pp. 642–51. DOI: 10.1007/978-3-642-36172 -2_200017.

Lopresti, Adrian L. (2017): "Curcumin for neuropsychiatric disorders: a review of in vitro, animal and human studies." In *Journal of Psychopharmacology* 31 (3), pp. 287–302. DOI: 10.1177/0269881116686883.

Saffron

Akhondzadeh Basti, Afshin; Moshiri, Esmail; Noorbala, Ahamad-Ali; Jamshidi, Amir-Hossein; Abbasi, Seyed Hesameddin; Akhondzadeh, Shahin (2007): "Comparison of petal of *Crocus sativus* L. and fluoxetine in the treatment of depressed outpatients: a pilot double-blind randomized trial." In *Progress in Neuro-Psychopharmacology & Biological Psychiatry* 31 (2), pp. 439–42. DOI: 10.1016/j.pnpbp.2006.11.010.

Moshiri, M.; Vahabzadeh, M.; Hosseinzadeh, H. (2015): "Clinical applications of saffron (*Crocus sativus*) and its constituents: a review." In *Drug Research* 65 (6), pp. 287–95. DOI: 10.1055/s-0034 -1375681.

Black Cohosh

Bai, Wenpei; Henneicke-von Zepelin, Hans-Heinrich; Wang, Shuyu; Zheng, Shurong; Liu, Jianli; Zhang, Zhonglan et al. (2007): "Efficacy and tolerability of a medicinal product containing an isopropanolic black cohosh extract in Chinese women with menopausal symptoms: a randomized, double blind, parallel-controlled study versus tibolone." In *Maturitas* 58 (1), pp. 31–41. DOI: 10.1016/j.maturitas.2007.04.009.

Nappi, Rossella E.; Malavasi, Barbara; Brundu, Benedetta; Facchinetti, Fabio (2005): "Efficacy of *Cimicifuga racemosa* on climacteric complaints: a randomized study versus low-dose transdermal estradiol." In *Gynecological Endocrinology* 20 (1), pp. 30–35.

Skullcap

Brock, Christine; Whitehouse, Julie; Tewfik, Ihab; Towell, Tony (2014): "American skullcap (*Scutellaria lateriflora*): a randomised, double-blind placebo-controlled crossover study of its effects on mood in healthy volunteers." In *Phytotherapy Research*: PTR 28 (5), pp. 692–98. DOI: 10.1002/ptr.5044.

Gasiorowski, Kazimierz; Lamer-Zarawska, Eliza; Leszek, Jerzy; Parvathaneni, Kalpana; Yendluri, Bharat Bhushan; Blach-Olszewska, Zofia; Aliev, Gjumrakch (2011): "Flavones from root of *Scutellaria baicalensis* Georgi: drugs of the future in neurodegeneration?" In *CNS & Neurological Disorders—Drug Targets* 10 (2), pp. 184–91.

Clary Sage

Lee, Kyung-Bok; Cho, Eun; Kang, Young-Sook (2014): "Changes in 5-hydroxytryptamine and cortisol plasma levels in menopausal women after inhalation of clary sage oil." In *Phytotherapy Research : PTR* 28 (11), pp. 1599–1605. DOI: 10.1002/ptr.5163.

Seol, Geun Hee; Shim, Hyun Soo; Kim, Pill-Joo; Moon, Hea Kyung; Lee, Ki Ho; Shim, Insop et al. (2010): "Antidepressant-like effect of *Salvia sclarea* is explained by modulation of dopamine activities in rats." In *Journal of Ethnopharmacology* 130 (1), pp. 187–90. DOI: 10.1016/j.jep.2010.04.035.

Chai Hu

Ushiroyama, Takahisa; Ikeda, Atsushi; Sakuma, Kou; Ueki, Minoru (2005): "Chai-hu-gui-zhi-gan-jiang-tang regulates plasma interleukin-6 and soluble interleukin-6 receptor concentrations and improves depressed mood in climacteric women with insomnia." In *The American Journal of Chinese Medicine* 33 (5), pp. 703–11. DOI: 10.1142/S0192415X05003338.

Rose

Conrad, Pam; Adams, Cindy (2012): "The effects of clinical aromatherapy for anxiety and depression in the high risk postpartum woman—a pilot study." In *Complementary Therapies in Clinical Practice* 18 (3), pp. 164–68. DOI: 10.1016/j.ctcp.2012.05.002.

Igarashi, Miho; Ikei, Harumi; Song, Chorong; Miyazaki, Yoshifumi (2014): "Effects of olfactory stimulation with rose and orange oil on prefrontal cortex activity." In *Complementary Therapies in Medicine* 22 (6), pp. 1027–31. DOI: 10.1016/j.ctim.2014.09.003.

Chapter 4

Sleep medicine

Wilt, Timothy J.; MacDonald, Roderick; Brasure, Michelle; Olson, Carin M.; Carlyle, Maureen; Fuchs, Erika et al. (2016): "Pharmacologic Treatment of Insomnia Disorder: An Evidence Report for a Clinical Practice Guideline by the American College of Physicians." In *Annals of Internal Medicine* 165 (2), pp. 103–112. DOI: 10.7326/M15-1781.

Lettuce

Yakoot, Mostafa; Helmy, Sherine; Fawal, Kamal (2011): "Pilot study of the efficacy and safety of lettuce seed oil in patients with sleep disorders." In *International Journal of General Medicine* 4, pp. 451–56. DOI: 10.2147/IJGM.S21529.

Lotus

Yan, Ming-Zhu; Chang, Qi; Zhong, Yu; Xiao, Bing-Xin; Feng, Li; Cao, Fang-Rui et al. (2015): "Lotus leaf alkaloid extract displays sedative-hypnotic and anxiolytic effects through GABAA receptor." In *Journal of Agricultural and Food Chemistry* 63 (42), pp. 9277–85. DOI: 10.1021/acs.jafc.5b04141.

Wuling

Lin, Yan; Wang, Xiao-yun; Ye, Ren; Hu, Wan-hua; Sun, Shu-chen; Jiao, Hong-juan et al. (2013): "Efficacy and safety of Wuling capsule, a single herbal formula, in Chinese subjects with insomnia: a multicenter, randomized, double-blind, placebo-controlled trial." In *Journal of Ethnopharmacology* 145 (1), pp. 320–27. DOI: 10.1016/j.jep.2012.11.009.

Ni, Xiaojia; Shergis, Johannah Linda; Guo, Xinfeng; Zhang, Anthony Lin; Li, Yan; Lu, Chuanjian; Xue, Charlie Changli (2015): "Updated clinical evidence of Chinese herbal medicine for insomnia: a systematic review and meta-analysis of randomized controlled trials." In *Sleep Medicine* 16 (12), pp. 1462–81. DOI: 10.1016/j.sleep.2015.08.012.

Mexican calea

Mayagoitia, L.; Díaz, J. L.; Contreras, C.M. (1986): "Psychopharmacologic analysis of an alleged oneirogenic plant: *Calea zacatechichi*." In *Journal of Ethnopharmacology* 18 (3), pp. 229–43.

Alpha-pinene

Yang, Hyejin; Woo, Junsung; Pae, Ae Nim; Um, Min Young; Cho, Nam-Chul; Park, Ki Duk et al. (2016): "α-Pinene, a major constituent of pine tree oils, enhances non-rapid eye movement sleep in mice through GABAA-benzodiazepine receptors."

In *Molecular Pharmacology* 90 (5), pp. 530–39. DOI: 10.1124/mol.116.105080.

Valerian

Fernández-San-Martin, Maria Isabel; Masa-Font, Roser; Palacios-Soler, Laura; Sancho-Gomez, Pilar; Calbo-Caldentey, Cristina; Flores-Mateo, Gemma (2010): "Effectiveness of valerian on insomnia: a meta-analysis of randomized placebo-controlled trials." In *Sleep Medicine* 11 (6), pp. 505–11. DOI: 10.1016/j.sleep.2009.12.009.

Poyares, Dalva R.; Guilleminault, Christian; Ohayon, Maurice M.; Tufik, Sergio (2002): "Can valerian improve the sleep of insomniacs after benzodiazepine withdrawal?" In *Progress in Neuro-Psychopharmacology & Biological Psychiatry* 26 (3), pp. 539–45.

Hop

Salter, Shanah; Brownie, Sonya (2010): "Treating primary insomnia—the efficacy of valerian and hops." In *Australian Family Physician* 39 (6), pp. 433–37.

Schmitz, M.; Jackel, M. (1998): "Comparative study for assessing quality of life of patients with exogenous sleep disorders (temporary sleep onset and sleep interruption disorders) treated with a hops-valerian preparation and a benzodiazepine drug." In *Wiener Medizinische Wochenschrift* (1998) 148 (13), pp. 291–98.

Chamomile

Howrey, Bret T.; Peek, M. Kristen; McKee, Juliet M.; Raji, Mukaila A.; Ottenbacher, Kenneth J.; Markides, Kyriakos S. (2016): "Chamomile consumption and mortality: a prospective study of Mexican origin older adults." In *The Gerontologist* 56 (6), pp. 1146–52. DOI: 10.1093/geront/gnv051.

Zick, Suzanna M.; Wright, Benjamin D.; Sen, Ananda; Arnedt, J. Todd (2011): "Preliminary examination of the efficacy and safety of a standardized chamomile extract for chronic primary insomnia: a randomized placebo-controlled pilot study." In *BMC Complementary and Alternative Medicine* 11, p. 78. DOI: 10.1186/1472-6882-11-78.

Jujube

Cao, Jie-Xin; Zhang, Qing-Ying; Cui, Su-Ying; Cui, Xiang-Yu; Zhang, Juan; Zhang, Yong-He et al. (2010): "Hypnotic effect of jujubosides from *Semen Ziziphi Spinosae*." In *Journal of Ethnopharmacology* 130 (1), pp. 163–66. DOI: 10.1016/j.jep.2010.03.023.

Ma, Yuan; Han, Huishan; Eun, Jae Soon; Kim, Hyoung Chun; Hong, Jin-Tae; Oh, Ki-Wan (2007): "Sanjoinine A isolated from Zizyphi Spinosi Semen augments pentobarbital-induced sleeping behaviors through the modification of GABA-ergic systems." In *Biological and Pharmaceutical Bulletin* 30 (9), pp. 1748–53.

Rodriguez Villanueva, Javier; Rodriguez Villanueva, Laura (2017): "Experimental and clinical pharmacology of *Ziziphus jujuba* Mill." In *Phytotherapy Research: PTR* 31 (3), pp. 347–65. DOI: 10.1002/ptr.5759.

California Poppy

Hanus, Michel; Lafon, Jacqueline; Mathieu, Marc (2004): "Double-blind, randomised, placebo-controlled study to evaluate the efficacy and safety of a fixed combination containing two plant extracts (*Crataegus oxyacantha and Eschscholtzia* [sic] *californica*) and magnesium in mild-to-moderate anxiety disorders." In *Current Medical Research and Opinion* 20 (1), pp. 63–71. DOI: 10.1185/030079903125002603.

Rolland, A.; Fleurentin, J.; Lanhers, M.C.; Misslin, R.; Mortier, F. (2001): "Neurophysiological effects of an extract of *Eschscholzia californica* Cham. (Papaveraceae)." In *Phytotherapy Research: PTR* 15 (5), pp. 377–81.

Tart Cherry

Garrido, M.; González-Gómez, D.; Lozano, M.; Barriga, C.; Paredes, S. D.; Rodriguez, A. B. (2013): "A Jerte valley cherry product provides beneficial effects on sleep quality: Influence on aging." In *The Journal of Nutrition, Health & Aging* 17 (6), pp. 553–60. DOI: 10.1007/s12603-013-0029-4.

Howatson, Glyn; Bell, Phillip G.; Tallent, Jamie; Middleton, Benita; McHugh, Malachy P.; Ellis,

Jason (2012): "Effect of tart cherry juice (*Prunus cerasus*) on melatonin levels and enhanced sleep quality." In *European Journal of Nutrition* 51 (8), pp. 909–16. DOI: 10.1007/s00394-011-0263-7.

Vervain

Khan, Abdul Waheed; Khan, Arif-Ullah; Ahmed, Touqeer (2016): "Anticonvulsant, anxiolytic, and sedative activities of *Verbena officinalis*." In *Frontiers in Pharmacology* 7, p.499. DOI: 10.3389/fphar.2016.00499.

Exercises

Archontogeorgis, K.; Nena, E.; Papanas, N.; Zissimopoulos, A.; Voulgaris, A.; Xanthoudaki, M.; et al. (2017): "Vitamin D levels in middle-aged patients with obstructive sleep apnoea syndrome." In *Current Vascular Pharmacology*. DOI: 10.2174/1570161115666170529085708.

Wang, Fang; Eun-Kyoung Lee, Othelia; Feng, Fan; Vitiello, Michael V.; Wang, Weidong; Benson, Herbert; et al. (2016): "The effect of meditative movement on sleep quality: A systematic review." In *Sleep Medicine Reviews* 30, pp. 43–52. DOI: 10.1016/j.smrv.2015.12.001.

Chapter 5

Butterbur

Agosti, R.; Duke, R. K.; Chrubasik, J. E.; Chrubasik, S. (2006): "Effectiveness of *Petasites hybridus* preparations in the prophylaxis of migraine: a systematic review." In *Phytomedicine* 13 (9–10), pp. 743–46. DOI: 10.1016/j.phymed.2006.02.008.

Lipton, R.B.; Göbel, H.; Einhäupl, K.M.; Wilks, K.; Mauskop, A. (2004): "*Petasites hybridus* root (butterbur) is an effective preventive treatment for migraine." In *Neurology* 63 (12), pp. 2240–44.

Osteoarthritis

Cameron, Melainie; Chrubasik, Sigrun (2014): "Oral herbal therapies for treating osteoarthritis." In *Cochrane Database of Systematic Reviews* (5), CD002947. DOI: 10.1002/14651858.CD002947.pub2.

Ernst, E. (2008): "Frankincense: systematic review." In *BMJ (Clinical Research Ed.)* 337, a2813.

Kratom

Swogger, Marc T.; Hart, Elaine; Erowid, Fire; Erowid, Earth; Trabold, Nicole; Yee, Kaila et al. (2015): "Experiences of kratom users: a qualitative analysis." In *Journal of Psychoactive Drugs* 47 (5), pp. 360–67. DOI: 10.1080/02791072.2015.1096434.

Cannabis

Williamson, E.M.; Evans, F.J. (2000): "Cannabinoids in clinical practice." In *Drugs* 60 (6), pp. 1303–14.

Rong, Carola; Lee, Yena; Carmona, Nicole E.; Cha, Danielle S.; Ragguett, Renee-Marie; Rosenblat, Joshua D. et al. (2017): "Cannabidiol in medical marijuana: research vistas and potential opportunities." In *Pharmacological Research* 121, pp. 213–18. DOI: 10.1016/j.phrs.2017.05.005.

Arnica

Iannitti, Tommaso; Morales-Medina, Julio César; Bellavite, Paolo; Rottigni, Valentina; Palmieri, Beniamino (2016): "Effectiveness and safety of *Arnica montana* in post-surgical setting, pain and inflammation." In *American Journal of Therapeutics* 23 (1), e184–97. DOI: 10.1097/MJT.0000000000000036.

Widrig, Reto; Suter, Andy; Saller, Reinhard; Melzer, Jörg (2007): "Choosing between NSAID and arnica for topical treatment of hand osteoarthritis in a randomised, double-blind study." In *Rheumatology International* 27 (6), pp. 585–91. DOI: 10.1007/s00296-007-0304-y.

Comfrey

Frost, R.; MacPherson, H.; O'Meara, S. (2013): "A critical scoping review of external uses of comfrey (*Symphytum* spp.)." In *Complementary Therapies in Medicine* 21 (6), pp. 724–45. DOI: 10.1016/j.ctim.2013.09.009.

Barna, Milos; Kucera, Alexander; Hladícova, Marie; Kucera, Miroslav (2007): "Der wundheilende Effekt einer Symphytum-Herba-Extrakt-Creme (*Symphytum* x *uplandicum* Nyman): Ergebnisse einer randomisierten, kontrollierten Doppelblindstudie." In *Wiener Medizinische Wochenschrift* (1946) 157 (21–22), pp. 569–74. DOI: 10.1007/s10354-007-0474-y.

Predel, H.G.; Giannetti, B.; Koll, R.; Bulitta, M.; Staiger, C. (2005): "Efficacy of a comfrey root extract ointment in comparison to a diclofenac gel in the treatment of ankle distortions: results of an observer-blind, randomized, multicenter study." In *Phytomedicine* 12 (10), pp. 707–14. DOI: 10.1016/j.phymed.2005.06.001.

Giannetti, B.M.; Staiger, C.; Bulitta, M.; Predel, H-G (2010): "Efficacy and safety of comfrey root extract ointment in the treatment of acute upper or lower back pain: results of a double-blind, randomised, placebo-controlled, multicenter trial." In *British Journal of Sports Medicine* 44 (9), pp. 637–41. DOI: 10.1136/bjsm.2009.058677.

Willow

Chrubasik, S.; Künzel, O.; Model, A.; Conradt, C.; Black, A. (2001): "Treatment of low back pain with a herbal or synthetic anti-rheumatic: a randomized controlled study. Willow bark extract for low back pain." In *Rheumatology* (Oxford, England) 40 (12), pp. 1388–93.

Desborough, Michael J.R.; Keeling, David M. (2017): "The aspirin story—from willow to wonder drug." In *British Journal of Haematology* 177 (5), pp. 674–83. DOI: 10.1111/bjh.14520.

Feverfew

Ernst, E.; Pittler, M.H. (2000): "The efficacy and safety of feverfew (*Tanacetum parthenium* L.): an update of a systematic review." In *Public Health Nutrition* 3 (4A), pp. 509–14.

Walking

O'Connor, S.R.; Tully, M.A.; Ryan, B; Bleakley, C.M.; Baxter, G.D.; Bradley, J.M.; McDonough, S.M. (2015): "Walking exercise for chronic musculoskeletal pain: systematic review and meta-analysis." In *Archives of Physical Medicine and Rehabilitation* 96 (4), pp. 724–34. e3. DOI: 10.1016/j.apmr.2014.12.003. Epub 2014 Dec 19.

Fokkenrood, Hugo J. P.; Bendermacher, Bianca L. W.; Lauret, Gert Jan; Willigendael, Edith M.; Prins, Martin H.; Teijink, Joep A. W. (2013): "Supervised exercise therapy versus non-supervised exercise therapy for intermittent claudication." In *The Cochrane Database of Systematic Reviews* (8), CD005263. DOI: 10.1002/14651858.CD005263.pub3.

Revord, L.P.; Lomond, K.V.; Loubert, P.V.; Hammer, R.L. (2016): "Acute effects of walking with Nordic poles in persons with mild to moderate low-back pain." In *International Journal of Exercise Science* 9 (4), pp. 507–13.

Yoo, W.G. (2017): "Effect of modified leg-raising exercise on the pain and pelvic angle of a patient with back pain and excessive lordosis." In *Journal of Physical Therapy Science* 29 (7), pp. 1281–82. DOI: 10.1589/jpts.29.1281.

Pain-Controlling Mindfulness

Brown, Melanie L.; Rojas, Enrique; Gouda, Suzanne (2017): "A mind-body approach to pediatric pain management." In *Children* (Basel, Switzerland) 4 (6). DOI: 10.3390/children4060050.

Till, Sara R.; Wahl, Heather N.; As-Sanie, Sawsan (2017): "The role of nonpharmacologic therapies in management of chronic pelvic pain: what to do when surgery fails." In *Current Opinion in Obstetrics & Gynecology* 29 (4), pp. 231–39. DOI: 10.1097/GCO.0000000000000376.

Chapter 6

Chinese angelica

Yeh, Tzu-Shao; Huang, Chi-Chang; Chuang, Hsiao-Li; Hsu, Mei-Chich (2014): "*Angelica sinensis* improves exercise performance and protects against physical fatigue in trained mice." In *Molecules* (Basel, Switzerland*)* 19 (4), pp. 3926–39. DOI: 10.3390/molecules19043926.

Snow Lotus

Lee, J.C.; Kao, J.Y.; Kuo, D.H.; Liao, C.F.; Huang, C.H.; Fan, L.L.; Way, T.D. (2011): "Antifatigue and antioxidant activity of alcoholic extract from *Saussurea involucrata*." In *Journal of Traditional and Complementary Medicine* 1 (1), pp. 64–68.

Bilberry

Matsunaga, N.; Imai, S.; Inokuchi, Y.; Shimazawa, M.; Yokota, S.; Araki, Y.; Hara, H. (2009): "Bilberry and its main constituents have neuroprotective effects against retinal neuronal damage in vitro and in vivo." In *Molecular Nutrition and Food Research* 53 (7), pp. 869–77. DOI: 10.1002/mnfr.200800394

Oak

Belcaro, G.; Cornelli, U.; Luzzi, R.; Ledda, A.; Cacchio, M.; Saggino, A.; Cesarone, MR.; Dugall, M.; Feragalli, B.; Hu, S.; Pellegrini, L.; Ippolito, E. (2015): "Robuvit® (Quercus robur extract) supplementation in subjects with chronic fatigue syndrome and increased oxidative stress. A pilot registry study." In *Journal of Neurosurgical Sciences* 59 (2), pp. 105–17.

Astragalus

Liu, Chung-Hsiang; Tsai, Chang-Hai; Li, Tsai-Chung; Yang, Yu-Wan; Huang, Wei-Shih; Lu, Ming-Kui et al. (2016): "Effects of the traditional Chinese herb Astragalus membranaceus in patients with poststroke fatigue: a double-blind, randomized, controlled preliminary study." In *Journal of Ethnopharmacology* 194, pp. 954–62. DOI: 10.1016/j.jep.2016.10.058.

Zhang, H.; Huang, J. (1990): "Preliminary study of traditional Chinese medicine treatment of minimal brain dysfunction: analysis of 100 cases." In *Zhong xi yi jie he za zhi* (*Chinese Journal of Modern Developments in Traditional Medicine*) 10 (5), pp. 278–79, 260.

Ginkgo

Gorby, Heather E.; Brownawell, Amy M.; Falk, Michael C. (2010): "Do specific dietary constituents and supplements affect mental energy? Review of the evidence." In *Nutrition Reviews* 68 (12), pp. 697–718. DOI: 10.1111/j.1753-4887.2010.00340.x.

Cieza, A.; Maier, P.; Pöppel, E. (2003): "Effects of *Ginkgo biloba* on mental functioning in healthy volunteers." *Archives of Medical Research* Volume 34, Issue 5 September–October 2003, pp. 373–81.

Zhang, Hong-Feng; Huang, Li-Bo; Zhong, Yan-Biao; Zhou, Qi-Hui; Wang, Hui-Lin; Zheng, Guo-Qing; Lin, Yan (2016): "An overview of systematic reviews of *Ginkgo biloba* extracts for mild cognitive impairment and dementia." In *Frontiers in Aging Neuroscience* 8, p. 276. DOI: 10.3389/fnagi.2016.00276.

Green Tea

White, David J.; de Klerk, Suzanne; Woods, William; Gondalia, Shakuntla; Noonan, Chris; Scholey, Andrew B. (2016): "Anti-stress, behavioral and magnetoencephalography effects of an L-theanine-based nutrient drink: a randomised, double-blind, placebo-controlled, crossover trial." In *Nutrients* 8 (1). DOI: 10.3390/nu8010053.

Yoto, Ai; Motoki, Mao; Murao, Sato; Yokogoshi, Hidehiko (2012): "Effects of L-theanine or caffeine intake on changes in blood pressure under physical and psychological stresses." In *Journal of Physiological Anthropology* 31, p.28. DOI: 10.1186/1880-6805-31-28.

Türközü, Duygu; Şanlier, Nevin (2017): "L-theanine, unique amino acid of tea, and its metabolism, health effects, and safety." In *Critical Reviews in Food Science and Nutrition* 57 (8), pp. 1681–87. DOI: 10.1080/10408398.2015.1016141.

Licorice

Guo, Jie; Yang, Chunxiao; Yang, Jiajia; Yao, Yang (2016): "Glycyrrhizic acid ameliorates cognitive impairment in a rat model of vascular dementia associated with oxidative damage and inhibition of voltage-gated sodium channels." In *CNS & Neurological Disorders—Drug Targets* 15 (8), pp. 1001–8.

Singh, Paramdeep; Singh, Damanpreet; Goel, Rajesh K. (2016): "Protective effect on phenytoin-induced cognition deficit in pentylenetetrazol kindled mice: a repertoire of *Glycyrrhiza glabra* flavonoid antioxidants." In *Pharmaceutical Biology* 54 (7), pp. 1209–18. DOI: 10.3109/13880209.2015.1063673.

Baschetti, R. (1995): "Liquorice and chronic fatigue syndrome." In *The New Zealand Medical Journal* 108 (1002), p. 259.

Garlic

Morihara, Naoaki; Nishihama, Takeshi; Ushijima, Mitsuyasu, Ide, Nagatoshi; Takeda, Hidekatsu; Hayama, Minoru (2007): "Garlic as an anti-fatigue agent." In *Molecular Nutrition & Food Research* 51 (11), pp. 1329–34. DOI: 10.1002/mnfr.200700062.

Morihara, Naoaki; Ushijima, Mitsuyasu; Kashimoto, Naoki; Sumioka, Isao; Nishihama, Takeshi; Hayama, Minoru; Takeda, Hidekatsu (2006): "Aged garlic extract ameliorates physical fatigue." In *Biological & Pharmaceutical Bulletin* 29 (5), pp. 962–66.

Nettle

Patel, Sita Sharan; Udayabanu, Malairaman (2014): "*Urtica dioica* extract attenuates depressive like behavior and associative memory dysfunction in dexamethasone induced diabetic mice." In *Metabolic Brain Disease* 29 (1), pp. 121–30. DOI: 10.1007/s11011-014-9480-0.

Toldy, Anna; Atalay, Mustafa; Stadler, Krisztián; Sasvári, Mária; Jakus, Judit; Jung, Kyung J. et al. (2009): "The beneficial effects of nettle supplementation and exercise on brain lesion and memory in rat." In *The Journal of Nutritional Biochemistry* 20 (12), pp. 974–81. DOI: 10.1016/j.jnutbio.2008.09.001.

Ginger

Molahosseini, A.; Taghavi, M. M.; Taghipour, Z.; Shabanizadeh, A.; Fatehi, F.; Kazemi Arababadi, M.; Eftekhar Vaghefe, S. H. (2016): "The effect of the ginger on the apoptosis of hippocampal cells according to the expression of BAX and Cyclin D1

genes and histological characteristics of brain in streptozotocin male diabetic rats." In *Cellular and Molecular Biology* 62 (12), pp. 1–5. DOI: 10.14715/cmb/2016.62.12.1.

Nakai, Megumi; Iizuka, Michiro; Matsui, Nobuaki; Hosogi, Kazuko; Imai, Akiko; Abe, Noriaki et al. (2016): "Bangle (*Zingiber purpureum*) improves spatial learning, reduces deficits in memory, and promotes neurogenesis in the dentate gyrus of senescence-accelerated mouse P8." In *Journal of Medicinal Food* 19 (5), pp. 435–41. DOI: 10.1089/jmf.2015.3562.

Matsui, Nobuaki; Kido, Yuki; Okada, Hideki; Kubo, Miwa; Nakai, Megumi; Fukuishi, Nobuyuki et al. (2012): "Phenylbutenoid dimers isolated from *Zingiber purpureum* exert neurotrophic effects on cultured neurons and enhance hippocampal neurogenesis in olfactory bulbectomized mice." In *Neuroscience Letters* 513 (1), pp. 72–77. DOI: 10.1016/j.neulet.2012.02.010.

Qi gong

Lee, Myeong Soo; Kim, Mo Kyung; Ryu, Hoon (2005): "Qi-training (qigong) enhanced immune functions: what is the underlying mechanism?" In *The International Journal of Neuroscience* 115 (8), pp. 1099–1104. DOI: 10.1080/00207450590914347.

Vera, Francisca M.; Manzaneque, Juan M.; Rodríguez, Francisco M.; Bendayan, Rebecca; Fernández, Nieves; Alonso, Antonio (2016): "Acute effects on the counts of innate and adaptive immune response cells after 1 month of Taoist qigong practice." In *International Journal of Behavioral Medicinev* 23 (2), pp. 198–203. DOI: 10.1007/s12529-015-9509-8.

Lucchetti, Giancarlo; de Oliveira, Renata Ferreira; Gonçalves, Juliane Piasseschi de Bernardin; Ueda, Suely Mitoi Ykko; Mimica, Lycia Mara Jenne; Lucchetti, Alessandra Lamas Granero (2013): "Effect of Spiritist 'passe' (Spiritual healing) on growth of bacterial cultures." In *Complementary Therapies in Medicine* 21 (6), pp. 627–32. DOI: 10.1016/j.ctim.2013.08.012.

Breathing

Hayama, Yuka; Inoue, Tomoko (2012): "The effects of deep breathing on 'tension-anxiety' and fatigue in cancer patients undergoing adjuvant chemotherapy." In *Complementary Therapies in Clinical Practice* 18 (2), pp. 94–98. DOI: 10.1016/j.ctcp.2011.10.001.

Goldstein, Michael R.; Lewis, Gregory F.; Newman, Ronnie; Brown, Janice M.; Bobashev, Georgiy; Kilpatrick, Lisa et al. (2016): "Improvements in well-being and vagal tone following a yogic breathing-based life skills workshop in young adults: two open-trial pilot studies." In *International Journal of Yoga* 9 (1), pp. 20–26. DOI: 10.4103/0973-6131.171718.

Carter, Kirtigandha Salwe; Carter, Robert (2016): "Breath-based meditation: a mechanism to restore the physiological and cognitive reserves for optimal human performance." In *World Journal of Clinical Cases* 4 (4), pp. 99–102. DOI: 10.12998/wjcc.v4.i4.99.

Chapter 7

Out of the box

Grundmann, Oliver (2017): "Patterns of kratom use and health impact in the US –results from an online survey." In *Drug and Alcohol Dependence* 176, pp. 63–70. DOI: 10.1016/j.drugalcdep.2017.03.007.

Ismail, Ismaliza; Wahab, Suzaily; Sidi, Hatta; Das, Srijit; Lin, Loo Jiann; Razali, Rosdinom (2017): "Kratom and future treatment for the opioids addiction and chronic pain: periculo beneficium?" In *Current Drug Targets*. DOI: 10.2174/1389450118666170425154120.

Engidawork, E. (2017): "Pharmacological and toxicological effects of *Catha edulis* F. (khat)." In *Phytotherapy Research* 31 (7), pp. 1019–28. DOI: 10.1002/ptr.5832.

Halpern, John H.; Sherwood, Andrea R.; Hudson, James I.; Yurgelun-Todd, Deborah; Pope, Harrison G. (2005): "Psychological and cognitive effects of long-term peyote use among Native Americans." In *Biological Psychiatry* 58 (8), pp. 624–31. DOI: 10.1016/j.biopsych.2005.06.038.

Chellian, Ranjithkumar; Pandy, Vijayapandi; Mohamed, Zahurin (2017): "Pharmacology and toxicology of α- and β-Asarone: a review of preclinical evidence." In *Phytomedicine* 32, pp. 41–58. DOI: 10.1016/j.phymed.2017.04.003.

Kiyofuji, Kana; Kurauchi, Yuki; Hisatsune, Akinori; Seki, Takahiro; Mishima, Satoshi; Katsuki, Hiroshi (2015): "A natural compound macelignan protects midbrain dopaminergic neurons from inflammatory degeneration via microglial arginase-1 expression." In *European Journal of Pharmacology* 760, pp. 129–35. DOI: 10.1016/j.ejphar.2015.04.021.

Parle, Milind; Dhingra, Dinesh; Kulkarni, S.K. (2004): "Improvement of mouse memory by *Myristica fragrans* seeds." In *Journal of Medicinal Food* 7 (2), pp. 157–61. DOI: 10.1089/1096620041224193.

Mind-Altering Brain States and Altered Neuronal Networks

Schartner, Michael M.; Carhart-Harris, Robin L.; Barrett, Adam B.; Seth, Anil K.; Muthukumaraswamy, Suresh D. (2017): "Increased spontaneous MEG signal diversity for psychoactive doses of ketamine, LSD and psilocybin." In *Scientific Reports* 7, p.46421. DOI: 10.1038/srep46421.

Tófoli, L.F.; de Araujo, D.B. (2016): "Treating addiction: perspectives from EEG and imaging studies on psychedelics." In *International Review of Neurobiology* 129, pp. 157–85. DOI: 10.1016/bs.irn.2016.06.005.

Sampedro, Frederic; de la Fuente Revenga, Mario; Valle, Marta; Roberto, Natalia; Domínguez-Clavé, Elisabet; Elices, Matilde et al. (2017): "Assessing the psychedelic 'after-glow' in ayahuasca users: post-acute neurometabolic and functional connectivity changes are associated with enhanced mindfulness capacities." In *The International Journal of Neuropsychopharmacology* 1;20 (9), pp. 698–711. DOI: 10.1093/ijnp/pyx036.

Citrus Fruits

Lamport, Daniel J.; Pal, Deepa; Macready, Anna L.; Barbosa-Boucas, Sofia; Fletcher, John M.; Williams, Claire M. et al. (2016): "The effects of flavanone-rich citrus juice on cognitive function and cerebral blood flow: an acute, randomised, placebo-controlled cross-over trial in healthy, young adults." In *The British Journal of Nutrition* 116 (12), pp. 2160–68. DOI: 10.1017 /S000711451600430X.

Sarubbo, F.; Ramis, M. R.; Kienzer, C.; Aparicio, S.; Esteban, S.; Miralles, A.; Moranta, D. (2017): "Chronic silymarin, quercetin and naringenin treatments increase monoamines synthesis and hippocampal SIRT1 levels improving cognition in aged rats." In *Journal of Neuroimmune Pharmacology*. DOI: 10.1007/s11481-017-9759-0.

Ruiz-Miyazawa, Kenji W.; Staurengo-Ferrari, Larissa; Mizokami, Sandra S.; Domiciano, Talita P.; Vicentini, Fabiana T.M.C.; Camilios-Neto, Doumit et al. (2017): "Quercetin inhibits gout arthritis in mice: induction of an opioid-dependent regulation of inflammasome." In *Inflammopharmacology*. DOI: 10.1007/s10787-017-0356-x.

Frankincense

Moussaieff, Arieh; Rimmerman, Neta; Bregman, Tatiana; Straiker, Alex; Felder, Christian C.; Shoham, Shai et al. (2008): "Incensole acetate, an incense component, elicits psychoactivity by activating TRPV3 channels in the brain." In *The FASEB Journal* 22 (8), pp. 3024–34. DOI: 10.1096 /fj.07-101865.

Hosseini-Sharifabad, Mohammad; Kamali-Ardakani, Razieh; Hosseini-Sharifabad, Ali (2016): "Beneficial effect of *Boswellia serrata* gum resin on spatial learning and the dendritic tree of dentate gyrus granule cells in aged rats." In *Avicenna Journal of Phytomedicine* 6 (2), pp. 189–97.

De Petrocellis, L.; Orlando, P.; Moriello, A.S.; Aviello, G.; Stott, C.; Izzo, A.A.; Di Marzo, V. (2012): "Cannabinoid actions at TRPV channels: effects on TRPV3 and TRPV4 and their potential relevance to gastrointestinal inflammation." *Acta Physiologica* (Oxford, England) 204 (2), pp. 255–66. DOI: 10.1111/j.1748-1716.

Mugwort

Deiml, T.; Haseneder, R.; Zieglgänsberger, W.; Rammes, G.; Eisensamer, B.; Rupprecht, R.; Hapfelmeier, G. (2004): "Alpha-thujone reduces 5-HT3 receptor activity by an effect on the agonist-reduced desensitization." In *Neuropharmacology* 46 (2), pp. 192–201.

Meschler, J.P.; Howlett, A.C. (1999): "Thujone exhibits low affinity for cannabinoid receptors but fails to evoke cannabimimetic responses." In *Pharmacology Biochemistry and Behavior* 62 (3), pp. 473–80.

He, Songming; Li, Lijun; Hu, Juying; Chen, Qiaoli; Shu, Weiqun (2015): "Effectiveness of traditional Chinese medicine (TCM) treatments on the cognitive functioning of elderly persons with mild cognitive impairment associated with white matter lesions." In *Shanghai Archives of Psychiatry* 27 (5), pp. 289–95. DOI: 10.11919/j.issn.1002-0829.215109.

Catnip

Hatch, R.C. (1972): "Effect of drugs on catnip (*Nepeta cataria*)-induced pleasure behavior in cats." In *American Journal of Veterinary Research* 33 (1), pp. 143–55.

Aydin, S.; Beis, R.; Oztürk, Y.; Baser, K.H.; Baser, C. (1998): "Nepetalactone: a new opioid analgesic from *Nepeta caesarea* Boiss." In *Journal of Pharmacy and Pharmacology* 50 (7), pp. 813–17.

Espín-Iturbe, Luz Teresa; López Yañez, Bernardo A.; Carrasco García, Apolo; Canseco-Sedano, Rodolfo; Vázquez-Hernández, Maribel; Coria-Avila, Genaro A. (2017): "Active and passive responses to catnip (*Nepeta cataria*) are affected by age, sex and early gonadectomy in male and female cats." In *Behavioral Processes* 142, pp. 110–15. DOI: 10.1016/j.beproc.2017.06.008.

Kolouri, Sepideh; Firoozabadi, Ali; Salehi, Alireza; Zarshenas, Mohammad M.; Dastgheib, Seyed Ali; Heydari, Mojtaba; Rezaeizadeh, Hossein (2016): "*Nepeta menthoides* Boiss. & Buhse freeze-dried aqueous extract versus sertraline in the treatment of major depression: a double-blind randomized controlled trial." In *Complementary Therapies*

in Medicine 26, pp. 164–70. DOI: 10.1016/j.ctim
.2016.03.016.

Absinthe

Russo, Ethan B. (2011): "Taming THC: potential
cannabis synergy and phytocannabinoid-
terpenoid entourage effects." In *British Journal
of Pharmacology* 163 (7), pp. 1344–64. DOI:
10.1111/j.1476-5381.2011.01238.x.

Czyzewska, Marta M.; Mozrzymas, Jerzy
W. (2013): "Monoterpene α-thujone exerts
a differential inhibitory action on GABA(A)
receptors implicated in phasic and tonic
GABAergic inhibition." In *European Journal of
Pharmacology* 702 (1–3), pp. 38–43. DOI: 10.1016/j.
ejphar.2013.01.032.

Deiml, T.; Haseneder, R.; Zieglgänsberger, W.;
Rammes, G.; Eisensamer, B.; Rupprecht, R.;
Hapfelmeier, G. (2004): "Alpha-thujone reduces
5-HT3 receptor activity by an effect on the agonist-
reduced desensitization." In *Neuropharmacology*
46 (2), pp. 192–201.

Wild Lettuce

Wesołowska, A.; Nikiforuk, A.; Michalska,
K.; Kisiel, W.; Chojnacka-Wójcik, E. (2006):
"Analgesic and sedative activities of lactucin
and some lactucin-like guaianolides in mice." In
Journal of Ethnopharmacology 107 (2), pp. 254–58.
DOI: 10.1016/j.jep.2006.03.003.

Yakoot, Mostafa; Helmy, Sherine; Fawal, Kamal
(2011): "Pilot study of the efficacy and safety of
lettuce seed oil in patients with sleep disorders."
In *International Journal of General Medicine* 4, pp.
451–56. DOI: 10.2147/IJGM.S21529.

Sayyah, Mohammad; Hadidi, Naghmeh;
Kamalinejad, Mohammad (2004): "Analgesic and
anti-inflammatory activity of Lactuca sativa seed
extract in rats." In *Journal of Ethnopharmacology*
92 (2–3), pp. 325–29. DOI: 10.1016/j.jep.2004.03.016.

Divine Sage

Cunningham, Christopher W.; Rothman,
Richard B.; Prisinzano, Thomas E. (2011):

"Neuropharmacology of the naturally occurring
kappa-opioid hallucinogen salvinorin A." In
Pharmacological Reviews 63 (2), pp. 316–47. DOI:
10.1124/pr.110.003244.

Addy, Peter H.; Garcia-Romeu, Albert; Metzger,
Matthew; Wade, Jenny (2015): "The subjective
experience of acute, experimentally-induced
Salvia divinorum inebriation." In *Journal of
Psychopharmacology* 29 (4), pp. 426–35. DOI:
10.1177/0269881115570081.

Taylor, George T.; Manzella, Francesca (2016):
"Kappa opioids, salvinorin A and major depressive
disorder." In *Current Neuropharmacology* 14 (2),
pp. 165–76.

Dos Santos, R.G.; Crippa, J.A.S.; Machado-de-
Sousa, J.P.; Hallak, J.E.C. (2014): "Salvinorin A
and related compounds as therapeutic drugs for
psychostimulant-related disorders." In *Current
Drug Abuse Reviews* 7 (2), pp. 128–32.

Chapter 8

Lavender

Kasper, Siegfried; Möller, Hans-Jürgen; Volz,
Hans-Peter; Schläfke, Sandra; Dienel, Angelika
(2017): "Silexan in generalized anxiety disorder:
investigation of the therapeutic dosage range
in a pooled data set." In *International Clinical
Psychopharmacology* 32 (4), pp. 195–204. DOI:
10.1097/YIC.0000000000000176.

Perry, R.; Terry, R.; Watson, L.K.; Ernst, E.
(2012): "Is lavender an anxiolytic drug? A
systematic review of randomized clinical trials." In
Phytomedicine 19 (8–9), pp. 825–35. DOI: 10.1016/j
.phymed.2012.02.013.

Lillehei, Angela Smith; Halcón, Linda L.; Savik,
Kay; Reis, Reilly (2015): "Effect of inhaled
lavender and sleep hygiene on self-reported sleep
issues: a randomized controlled trial." In *Journal
of Alternative and Complementary Medicine*
(New York, N.Y.) 21 (7), pp. 430–38. DOI: 10.1089/
acm.2014.0327.

López, Víctor; Nielsen, Birgitte; Solas, Maite;
Ramírez, Maria J.; Jäger, Anna K. (2017):

"Exploring pharmacological mechanisms of lavender (*Lavandula angustifolia*) essential oil on central nervous system targets." In *Frontiers in Pharmacology* 8, p.280. DOI: 10.3389/fphar.2017 .00280.

Kasper, Siegfried; Müller, Walter E.; Volz, Hans-Peter; Möller, Hans-Jürgen; Koch, Egon; Dienel, Angelika (2017): "Silexan in anxiety disorders: Clinical data and pharmacological background." In *The World Journal of Biological Psychiatry*, pp. 1–9. DOI: 10.1080/15622975.2017.1331046.

Lemon Balm

Shakeri, Abolfazl; Sahebkar, Amirhossein; Javadi, Behjat (2016): "*Melissa officinalis* L.—a review of its traditional uses, phytochemistry and pharmacology." In *Journal of Ethnopharmacology* 188, pp. 204–28. DOI: 10.1016/j.jep.2016.05.010.

Gromball, Jürgen; Beschorner, Frank; Wantzen, Christian; Paulsen, Ute; Burkart, Martin (2014): "Hyperactivity, concentration difficulties and impulsiveness improve during seven weeks' treatment with valerian root and lemon balm extracts in primary school children." In *Phytomedicine* 21 (8–9), pp. 1098–1103. DOI: 10.1016/j.phymed.2014.04.004.

Huang, L.; Abuhamdah, S.; Howes, M.J.; Dixon, C.L.; Elliot, M.S.; Ballard, C.; Holmes, C.; Burns, A.; Perry, E.K.; Francis, P.T.; Lees, G.; Chazot, P.L. (2008): "Pharmacological profile of essential oils derived from *Lavandula angustifolia* and *Melissa officinalis* with anti-agitation properties: focus on ligand-gated channels." In *Journal of Pharmacy and Pharmacology* 60 (11), pp. 1515–22. DOI: 10.1211/jpp/60.11.0013. Erratum in *Journal of Pharmacy and Pharmacology* 2009 61 (2), p.267. Dixon, Christine L [added]. PMID:18957173

Roseroot

Darbinyan, V.; Aslanyan, G.; Amroyan, E.; Gabrielyan, E.; Malmström, C.; Panossian, A. (2007): "Clinical trial of *Rhodiola rosea* L. extract SHR-5 in the treatment of mild to moderate depression." In *Nordic Journal of Psychiatry* 61 (5), pp. 343–48. DOI: 10.1080/08039480701643290.

Darbinyan, V.; Kteyan, A.; Panossian, A.; Gabrielian, E.; Wikman, G.; Wagner, H. (2000): "*Rhodiola rosea* in stress induced fatigue—a double-blind cross-over study of a standardized extract SHR-5 with a repeated low-dose regimen on the mental performance of healthy physicians during night duty." In *Phytomedicine* 7 (5), pp. 365–71. DOI: 10.1016/S0944-7113(00)80055-0.

Panossian, A.; Wagner, H. (2005): "Stimulating effect of adaptogens: an overview with particular reference to their efficacy following single dose administration." In *Phytotherapy Research: PTR* 19 (10), pp. 819–38. DOI: 10.1002/ptr.1751.

Ishaque, Sana; Shamseer, Larissa; Bukutu, Cecilia; Vohra, Sunita (2012): "*Rhodiola rosea* for physical and mental fatigue: a systematic review." In *BMC Complementary and Alternative Medicine* 12, p. 70. DOI: 10.1186/1472-6882-12-70.

Cropley, Mark; Banks, Adrian P.; Boyle, Julia (2015): "The effects of *Rhodiola rosea* L. extract on anxiety, stress, cognition and other mood symptoms." In *Phytotherapy Research : PTR* 29 (12), pp. 1934–39. DOI: 10.1002/ptr.5486.

Ginseng

Vogler, B.K.; Pittler, M.H.; Ernst, E. (1999): "The efficacy of ginseng. A systematic review of randomized clinical trials." In *European Journal of Clinical Pharmacology* 55 (8), pp. 567–75.

Sørensen, Henrik; Sonne, Jesper (1996): "A double-masked study of the effects of ginseng on cognitive functions." In *Current Therapeutic Research* 57 (12), pp. 959–68. DOI: 10.1016/S0011-393X(96)80114-7.

Ossoukhova, A.; Owen, L.; Savage, K.; Meyer, M.; Ibarra, A.; Roller, M.; Pipingas, A.; Wesnes, K.; Scholey, A. (2015): "Improved working memory performance following administration of a single dose of American ginseng (*Panax quinquefolius* L.) to healthy middle-age adults." In *Human Psychopharmacology* 30 (2), pp. 108–22. DOI: 10.1002/hup.2463. PMID:25778987

Chen, X.; Zhou, M.; Li, Q.;Yang, J.; Zhang, Y.; Zhang, D.; Kong, S.; Zhou, D.; He, L. (2008): "Sanchi for acute ischaemic stroke." In *Cochrane*

Database of Systematic Reviews 8 (4) : CD006305. DOI: 10.1002/14651858.CD006305.pub2.

Kennedy, D.O.; Scholey, A.B.; Wesnes, K.A. (2001): "Differential, dose dependent changes in cognitive performance following acute administration of a *Ginkgo biloba*/*Panax ginseng* combination to healthy young volunteers." In *Nutritional Neuroscience* 4 (5), pp. 399–412.

Kim, Young-Sook; Woo, Jung-Yoon; Han, Chang-Kyun; Chang, Il-Moo (2015): "Safety analysis of *Panax ginseng* in randomized clinical trials. A systematic review." In *Medicines* 2 (2), pp. 106–26. DOI: 10.3390/medicines2020106.

Vogler, B.K.; Pittler, M.H.; Ernst, E. (1999): "The efficacy of ginseng: A systematic review of randomized clinical trials." In *European Journal of Clinical Pharmacology* 55 (8), pp. 567–75.

Ahmed, Touqeer; Raza, Syed Hammad; Maryam, Afifa; Setzer, William N.; Braidy, Nady; Nabavi, Seyed Fazel et al. (2016): "Ginsenoside Rb1 as a neuroprotective agent: A review." In *Brain Research Bulletin* 125, pp. 30–43. DOI: 10.1016/j.brainresbull.2016.04.002.

Cocoa

Scholey, A.; Owen, L. (2013): "Effects of chocolate on cognitive function and mood: a systematic review." *Nutrition Reviews* 71 (10), pp. 665–81. DOI: 10.1111/nure.12065.

Larsson, S.C.; Virtamo, J.; Wolk, A. (2012): "Chocolate consumption and risk of stroke: a prospective cohort of men and meta-analysis." *Neurology* 79 (12), pp. 1223–29. DOI: 10.1212/WNL.ob013e31826aacfa.

Sansone, Roberto; Ottaviani, Javier I.; Rodriguez-Mateos, Ana; Heinen, Yvonne; Noske, Dorina; Spencer, Jeremy P.; et al. (2017): "Methylxanthines enhance the effects of cocoa flavanols on cardiovascular function: randomized, double-masked controlled studies." In *The American Journal of Clinical Nutrition* 105 (2), pp. 352–60. DOI: 10.3945/ajcn.116.140046.

Smit, Hendrik J.; Gaffan, Elizabeth A.; Rogers, Peter J. (2004): "Methylxanthines are the psycho-pharmacologically active constituents of chocolate." In *Psychopharmacology* 176 (3–4), pp. 412–19. DOI: 10.1007/s00213-004-1898-3.

Forest bathing

Park BJ, Tsunetsugu Y, Kasetani T, Kagawa T, Miyazaki Y. (2010): "The physiological effects of Shinrin-yoku (taking in the forest atmosphere or forest bathing): evidence from field experiments in 24 forests across Japan." *Environmental Health and Preventive Medicine*. 2010;15(1):18-26. DOI:10.1007/s12199-009-0086-9.

The Future for Medicinal Plants and Herbs

Adaptogens

Panossian, Alexander (2017): "Understanding adaptogenic activity: specificity of the pharmacological action of adaptogens and other phytochemicals" In *Annals of the New York Academy of Sciences*. DOI: 10.1111/nyas.13399.

Panossian, Alexander G. (2013): "Adaptogens in mental and behavioral disorders." In *The Psychiatric Clinics of North America* 36 (1), pp. 49–64. DOI: 10.1016/j.psc.2012.12.005.

Haidan Yuan; Qianqian Ma; Heying Cui; Guancheng Lui; Xiaoyan Zhao; Wei Li; Guangchun Piao (2017): "How can synergism of traditional medicines benefit from network pharmacology?" *Molecules*. 2017 Jul 7;22(7). pii: E1135. DOI: 10.3390/molecules22071135.

Epigenetics

Dauncey, M. J. (2014): "Nutrition, the brain and cognitive decline: insights from epigenetics." In *European Journal of Clinical Nutrition* 68 (11), pp. 1179–85. DOI: 10.1038/ejcn.2014.173.

Moore, David Scott (2015): *The Developing Genome: An Introduction to Behavioral Epigenetics*. New York, NY: Oxford University Press.

Denhardt, David T. (2017): "Effect of stress on human biology: Epigenetics, adaptation, inheritance, and social significance." In *Journal of Cellular Physiology*. DOI: 10.1002/jcp.25837.

Sharma, Abhay (2017): "Transgenerational epigenetics: Integrating soma to germline communication with gametic inheritance." In *Mechanisms of Aging and Development* 163, pp. 15–22. DOI: 10.1016/j.mad.2016.12.015.

Xue, Jing; Schoenrock, Sarah A.; Valdar, William; Tarantino, Lisa M.; Ideraabdullah, Folami Y. (2016): "Maternal vitamin D depletion alters DNA methylation at imprinted loci in multiple generations." In *Clinical Epigenetics* 8, p. 107. DOI: 10.1186/s13148-016-0276-4.

Choi, Chang Soon; Gonzales, Edson Luck; Kim, Ki Chan; Yang, Sung Min; Kim, Ji-Woon; Mabunga, Darine Froy et al. (2016): "The transgenerational inheritance of autism-like phenotypes in mice exposed to valproic acid during pregnancy." In *Scientific Reports* 6, p. 36250. DOI: 10.1038/srep36250.

Further Relevant Publications by the Authors

Howes, Melanie-Jayne R.; Perry, Nicolette S. L.; Houghton, Peter J. (2003): "Plants with traditional uses and activities, relevant to the management of Alzheimer's disease and other cognitive disorders." In *Phytotherapy Research: PT*R 17 (1), pp. 1–18. DOI: 10.1002/ptr.1280.

Perry, Elaine; Howes, Melanie-Jayne R. (2011): "Medicinal plants and dementia therapy: herbal hopes for brain aging?" In *CNS Neuroscience & Therapeutics* 17 (6), pp. 683–98. DOI: 10.1111/j.1755-5949.2010.00202.x.

Howes, Melanie-Jayne R.; Perry, Elaine (2011): "The role of phytochemicals in the treatment and prevention of dementia." In *Drugs & Aging* 28 (6), pp. 439–68. DOI: 10.2165/11591310-000000000-00000.

Perry, Nicolette; Perry, Elaine (2006): "Aromatherapy in the management of psychiatric disorders: clinical and neuropharmacological perspectives." In *CNS Drugs* 20 (4), pp. 257–80.

Perry, N.S.L.; Menzies, R.; Hodgson, F.; Wedgewood, P.; Howes, M-J.R.; Brooker, H.J.; Wesnes, K.A.; Perry, E.K. (2017): "A randomised double-blind placebo-controlled pilot trial of a combined extract of sage, rosemary and melissa, traditional herbal medicines, on the enhancement of memory in normal healthy subjects, including influence of age." *Phytomedicine* 39, pp. 42–48. DOI: 10.1016/j.phymed.2017.08.015.

Index

Page numbers in *italics* indicate pictures.

crocin, 44, 77

Crocus sativus (saffron), 4, 44, *66*, 76–77, 194, 216

Culpeper, Nicholas, 36, 51, 128

cumin (*Cuminum cyminum*), 44, 74

Curcuma longa (turmeric), 5, 74–76, 118, 150, 164, 216

curcumin, 5, 75–76

cure-alls. *See* panaceas

curry recipe, 74

Cytisus scoparius (broom), 162

D

daffodil (*Narcissus pseudonarcissus*), 40, 41

dark chocolate, 68, 196–97

David Geffen School of Medicine, 60

dementia, 17–19, 40–41, 85, 114, 159, 183, 188. *See also* cognition boosters

depression relievers. *See* blues busters

De Quincey, Thomas, 91

devil's claw, 118

diabetes, 26, 52, 61, 75

dill (*Anethum graveolens*), 117

Dilston Physic Garden, *5–7*, *17–19*, 41, 51, 114, 127, 150, 158–60

dimethyltryptamine (DMT), 70, 162, 164–65

Dioscorides, 24, 96, 108, 148, 152, 172, 184, 190

divine sage (*Salvia divinorum*), 51, 113, 160–61, 173–75, 225

dog rose (*Rosa canina*), 86–87

dopamine, 69–70, 77, 91, 121, 164, 203

dreams, 91–93, 95, 103–4, 109, 169

drink recipes. *See* recipes

E

Eastern walnut (*Juglans regia*), 59–60

Echium amoenum (red feathers), *69*

elderly persons, 24, 40–41, 51, 53, 145, 193, 196. *See also* Alzheimer's disease; dementia

Eleutherococcus senticosus (Siberian ginseng), 191, 193, 200

endorphins, 17, 78, 112–13, 203

energizers

overview, 136–43

astragalus, 137, 144–45, 146, 221

caffeine, 4, 5, 85, 100, 139–40, 147–48

cocoa, 137, *138*, 180, *183*, 195–97, 227

folklore on, 144, 145, 147, 148, 151, 152, 154

garlic, 109, 150–52, 222

ginger, 44, 74, 118, *136*, 146, 149–50, 154–55, 222

ginkgo, 145–46, 154, 194, 221

ginseng, *137*, 180, *182*–83, 193–95, 200, 226–27

green tea, 3, 69, 113, 147–48, 221

licorice, 146, 148–49, 221

nettle, *139*, 150, 152–53, 222

research on, 140, 144–45, 147–48, 151–53, 154

roseroot, 44, 178, 180, 190–92, 200

epigenetics, 200–201

Equisetum arvense (horsetail), 117

Eschscholzia californica (California poppy), *17*, 107–8, 218

essential oils, 203–4

bergamot, 34–36, 164–65, 213

for breathing exercises, 56, 149, 155

chamomile, 101–3, 218

in citrus spray, 165

clary sage, 84–85, 216–17

in cleaning spray, 47

Dilston's research on, 17–19

in face cream, 73, 167

frankincense, 166–67, 224

lavender, 69, 101, 184–85

neroli, 29–31, 102, 164

peppermint, 52, 56, 58–59, 121

rose, 84, 86–87, 217

rosemary, 52, 54–56, 215

European oak (*Quercus robur*), 137, 140, *141*

European sage (*Salvia officinalis*), 4, 10, *11*, 41, 51–52, 214–15

exercise, benefits of, 32, 52, 102, 104, 143, 155, 19

F

face cream, 73, 167

fatigue fighters. *See* energizers

fennel (*Foeniculum vulgare*), 20, 21, 74, 172, 188

vitality. *See* energizers

Vitis labrusca (Concord grape), 44

Vitis vinifera (grape), *113*

W

walking, benefits of, 41, 122, 186

walnut (*Juglans*), 34, 59–60, 62, 215

white sage (*Salvia apiana*), 168

white willow (*Salix alba*), 113, 114, 130–31, 132, 133, 220

wild lettuce (*Lactuca virosa*), 93, 94, 97, 172–73, 225

willow bark, 114, 126, 130–31, 220

Withania somnifera (ashwagandha), 17, 24–25, 93, 137, 180, 213

wormwood (*Artemisia absinthium*), 171–72

wuling, 94–95, 217

Y

yangonin, 23

ylang-ylang (*Cananga odorata*), 58, *93*

yoga, 32, 102, 104. *See also* breathing techniques

yueju, 69

Z

Zingiber officinale (ginger), 44, 74, 118, *136*, 146, 149–50, 154–55, 222

Ziziphus jujuba (jujube), 44, 103–4, 218

Acknowledgments

In the preparation of this book we are indebted to Anna Mumford, who has helped us transform information from our workshops on Botanic Brain Boosters in the Northeast of England into a book for global readership, and to both Robert Forster and Bob Logan for helping with the writing. Our interest and research into plants for the brain has depended on many colleagues with whom we have carried out medicinal plant research over the last twenty years, including Professor Clive Ballard, Professor Paul Francis, Professor Peter Houghton, Dr. Melanie Howes, Professor Peter Jenner, Ross Menzies, Professor Elizabeta Mukaetova-Ladinska, Dr. Edward Okello, Professor Robert Perry, Dr. Sergey Savelev, Professor Andrew Scholey, Dr. George Wake, and Professor Keith Wesnes.

NP and EP

Picture Acknowledgments

CC BY 3.0 via Wikimedia Commons/Luis Nunes Alberto https://commons.wikimedia.org/wiki/ File%3ALactuca_virosa.jpg 180

David Taylor 16-17, 76, 99, 126

Garden World Images 93

istock.com/FurmanAnna 150-1

Oliver Fowler 240

Shutterstock.com/Africa Studio 108, Alexander Raths 102, Alexey Stiop 127, Anastasila Malinich 149, Apple's Eye Studio 64-5, Augusto809 201, Blueeyes 189, Boonchuay1970 83, chenzhang 56-7, CrispyPork 100, de2marco 115, Del Boy 53, 186, Diana Mower 139, domnitskey 44, Doug Stacey 181, dvoevnore 166, Elementals 103, emberiza 179, Enlightened Media 30, Fresnei 74, g215 160, GoncharukMaks 172, Goran Bogicevic 77, gresei 203, gyu sik 190, haraldmuc 177, Henrik Larsson 175, Hortimages 192, Igor Cheri 145, Inga_Ivanova 52, JPC-PROD 20, Julia Sudnitskaya 147, Kaiskynet Studio 43, Katarzyna Mazurowska 168, Kati Finell 71, Kazakov Maksim 104, Kostrez 10 , Krungchingplxs 101, krutar 35, Laszlo Halasi 130-1, LAURA_VN 155, Le Do 58, Linda George 78-79, LutsenkoLarissa 28, lzf 29, Madlen 32, Manfred Ruckszio 75, 87, 138, Marako85 121, Maren Winter 50, Margrit Hirsch 67, marilyn barbone 54, Markos Loizou 123, Maryna Pleshkun 148, Maximuit 169, michajela 106-7, Nattika 69, NatUlrich 113, Nella 94, Nenov Brothers Images 133, 140, nevodka 128, ninoninos 124, Nyvlt-art 33, Only Fabrizio 162, petelin 49, Peter Paunchev 194-5, Phototy 144, picturepartners 136, 167, Pixeljoy 152, PJ photography 48, puchkovo48 26, Ratmaner 109, Robert Przybysz 21, Robin W 171, Rostislav Ageev 191, roundstripe 174, saiko3p 146, Sann von mai 38, Sarah2 188, SasinTipchai 40-41, Scisetti Alfio 59, 61, 80, 132, 196, SK Herb 156, Sonja C 120, spline_x 92, 116, 198, Starover Sibiriak 122, 125, Studio Grand Ouest 86, Sumikophoto 25, svrid79 88, Tim UR 62, 114, Tunedin by Westend61 66, Vaclav Mach 98, Valentina Razumova 84, valvirga 19, Vishnevskly Vasily 12, Vitalii Kazannyk 24, Volosina 111, 153, Wavebreakmedia 18, Workretro 159

Terry Walsh 13, 14, 15,27

About the Authors

Nicolette Perry has a PhD in pharmacognosy from King's College London and has researched and published on medicinal plants for the brain. Her research into sage for Alzheimer's disease triggered a move to research central nervous system plants at Newcastle University. Her long-term interest, beginning with a degree in biology on health and disease, is in the science behind the use of plants for health, with a particular focus on aromatic plants for the brain. She is director of Dilston Physic Garden, now a nonprofit established for education in medicinal plants, where she runs workshops, organizes talks on plants for health, and teaches on the Foundation in Plant Medicine. She is keen to convey the science behind plants as herbal medicines, particularly for their preventative role and as an adjunct to mainstream medicine. She also enjoys spending time with her British artist husband and two children, walking, reading, and cooking outdoors.

Elaine Perry is emeritus professor of neuroscience at Newcastle University and founder and curator of Dilston Physic Garden. She has written and contributed to numerous scientific articles and books on topics that include Alzheimer's disease and autism, medicinal plants for cognition and mood, and consciousness including visual hallucinations. Dilston Physic Garden began as a place to grow and research the properties of certain plants in relation to memory loss and dementia. Positive results followed from laboratory testing, and Dilston has become known as a place that brings together the worlds of alternative therapies and orthodox medicine. Elaine also enjoys playing the piano, visiting her Scottish homeland, and exploring the subject of consciousness in theoretical (conceptual) and practical (meditative) ways.